T0202008

Immigration, Cultural Identity, and Mental Health

Immigration, Cultural Identity, and Mental Health

Psycho-social Implications of the Reshaping of America

EUGENIO M. ROTHE, M.D.
PROFESSOR OF PSYCHIATRY AND BEHAVIORAL HEALTH
HERBERT WERTHEIM COLLEGE OF MEDICINE
ADJUNCT PROFESSOR
LATIN AMERICAN AND CARIBBEAN CENTER AND
THE CUBAN RESEARCH INSTITUTE
FLORIDA INTERNATIONAL UNIVERSITY
MIAMI, FL

ANDRES J. PUMARIEGA, M.D.
PROFESSOR AND CHIEF
DIVISION OF CHILD AND ADOLESCENT PSYCHIATRY
DEPARTMENT OF PSYCHIATRY
UNIVERSITY OF FLORIDA COLLEGE OF
MEDICINE AND UF HEALTH
GAINESVILLE, FL

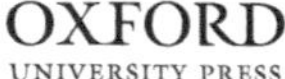

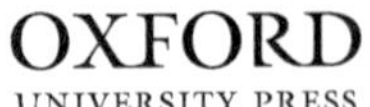

Oxford University Press is a department of the University of Oxford. It furthers the University's objective of excellence in research, scholarship, and education by publishing worldwide. Oxford is a registered trade mark of Oxford University Press in the UK and certain other countries.

Published in the United States of America by Oxford University Press
198 Madison Avenue, New York, NY 10016, United States of America.

Library of Congress Cataloging-in-Publication Data
Names: Rothe, Eugenio M., author. | Pumariega, Andres J., author.
Title: Immigration, cultural identity, and mental health /
Eugenio M. Rothe, M.D., Andres J. Pumariega, M.D.
Description: New York, NY : Oxford University Press, [2020] |
Includes bibliographical references and index.
Identifiers: LCCN 2019043009 (print) | LCCN 2019043010 (ebook) |
ISBN 9780190661700 (hardback) | ISBN 9780190661724 (epub) |
ISBN 9780190929466 (online) | ISBN 9780190929459 (oso)
Subjects: LCSH: Immigrants—Mental health—United States. |
Cultural psychiatry—United States. | Emigration and
immigration—Psychological aspects.
Classification: LCC RC451.4.E45 R68 2020 (print) | LCC RC451.4.E45 (ebook) |
DDC 362.2086/912—dc23
LC record available at https://lccn.loc.gov/2019043009
LC ebook record available at https://lccn.loc.gov/2019043010

9 8 7 6 5 4 3 2 1

Printed by Integrated Books International, United States of America

We dedicate this book with gratitude to our American wives, Anne and JoAnne and to our Hispanic-American children, Galicia and Miguel, and Cristina and Nicole, so they will continue their quest of making this a better world.

CONTENTS

FOREWORD

Immigration, Cultural Identity, and Mental Health is a unique book because it defines culture and identity from a developmental perspective, therefore delving more deeply into the psychological, social, and biological aspects of the immigrant and refugee experience in the United States of America. It explains how these experiences help to shape the development of the person's cultural identity. The book presents a very detailed discussion of the concept of *acculturation* and reviews all of the available literature on the subject. It also covers the sociological, anthropological, political, and economic aspects of the immigrant and refugee experience and how these variables impact mental health, thus presenting the experience of migration from a very broad and humanistic perspective. This book embarks on a deep exploration of the *psychodynamic experience of immigration* while covering the epidemiological risk factors and protective factors related to the immigrant experience. It thus presents ample and up-to-date empirically based data.

The book has a unique chapter addressing the true and accurate statistics of *immigrant criminality* and explores and analyzes these data under a new lens, helping to dispel the myths that result from contemporary anti-immigrant rhetoric. It also explains the types of crimes committed by immigrants, immigrants as victims of crime, cultural crimes, and motivations; it provides explanatory narratives presented by those who violate immigration laws. In addition, it covers the history of immigrant criminality in the United States.

The book has another important chapter addressing *immigrant narratives* and the role and importance of the personal–historical narrative in life story construction and the narrative as a therapeutic tool that can help to repair the trauma of loss and dislocation suffered by many immigrants when they leave their country of origin and begin a life in a new host country. It also introduces the role of the *new immigrant narratives* in contemporary literature and how this literature can be used by teachers and parents to help integrate the experiences of the different generations of the immigrant family. It can also be used to educate the younger generations of Americans about the country's new cultural diversity.

There is a chapter that explains the new concept of *transnational identities* that result from the improved communication technologies as well as from more accessible travel, both of which have deeply changed the immigrant experience and are part of the new phenomenon of globalization. Another interesting chapter analyzes the phenomenon of *return migrations* comparing the points of view of the returning immigrant with those of the ones who stayed behind, further analyzing this topic from a psychological and socioeconomic perspective. It also explains the psychological meaning of *pilgrimages*, in which the pilgrim does not necessarily visit the land of his or her actual birth or upbringing, but the land of the ancestral family history in an attempt to bridge the gaps between the generations and to better integrate the pilgrim's sense of ethnic and cultural identity.

In addition, this book has an extensive and well-documented chapter on the refugee experience, outlining the current worldwide refugee crisis and explaining the sociopolitical reasons behind the crisis. It offers new evidence-based treatments for this population.

This is a very comprehensive and well-written book that covers adults, children, adolescents, and families and describes the sociocultural experience of the various generations of immigrants in their adaptation to life in the United States. It also explores the *immigration-related family separations* as well as the psychological impact faced by the children who stay behind and later reunify with their parents in the United States. Those families separated by deportation are mentioned.

Finally, the book presents a comprehensive chapter on *culturally sensitive and culturally competent evidence-based mental health treatments* for the various generations of these populations, including recommendations on ethnopharmacology.

One of the many strengths of the book is the very compelling and clearly explained clinical cases, which help to illustrate the theoretical concepts that are presented in each chapter.

This book is a very timely and very valuable contribution to the bio-psycho-social study of the immigrant experience pertaining to the United States in its first generation and beyond. It is an essential tool for students and professionals in the social sciences; in the fields of social work, psychology, medicine, and psychiatry; and for members of government organizations responsible for urban planning, policy, and budgets, as well as for agencies dealing with the reception of, placement of, and assistance provided to immigrants and refugees.

Pedro Ruiz, M.D.
Professor of Psychiatry
Baylor Medical College of Medicine
Houston, Texas
Past President, American Psychiatric Association
Past President, World Psychiatric Association

PREFACE

The United States accepts the highest percentage of immigrants and refugees of any nation on Earth, and in the United States today, with the exception of Native Americans, the great majority of Americans either are immigrants or are descended from an immigrant.

Until the mid-twentieth century, the United States received predominantly European immigrants, whose racial and cultural characteristics came to define the ethnicity of the mainstream American culture, but in the past 40 years, non-European immigration has increased. By the year 2050, European-origin Americans will no longer be the numerical majority. This rapidly changing demographic landscape, characterized by an increasing multiracial and multicultural population is a result of three major factors: (1) the progressive aging and low birth rate of its European-origin population; (2) the lower mean ages and increasing birth rates in non-European minority groups; and (3) a significant increase in immigration from Latin America, Asia, and Africa.

These new growing populations are diverse in their racial, ethnic, and national origin, in their migration characteristics, and in their socioeconomic makeup. As a group, they are different from the older, European-origin, White, and higher socioeconomic mainstream population. Poverty, violence, wars, and political turmoil continue to ravage many countries around the world today, and this has resulted in large numbers of immigrants arriving to the shores of the more affluent countries with healthier economies and political stability. In many of these host countries, there is already a visible trend in which some of the citizens retreat to their traditional–cultural values and beliefs out of fear that those cultures and their adherents will become extinct or that they will be overwhelmed by growing groups of "others" in their midst.

Since our origins as a species, beginning in the Lower Paleolithic about 3.3 million years ago and into the Bronze Age approximately 6,500 years ago, early humans lived in small family groups of *hunter–gatherers,* probably traveled only a few miles away from their place of birth, and rarely encountered other groups different from themselves. These early hunter–gatherers developed a series of beliefs, behaviors, and traditions that allowed them to survive and to evolve into the modern humans of the present day. Among these beliefs are as follows: (1) The first is *ethnocentrism,* or the belief that their group is the center of the universe, and that they are the right ones. (2) *The need to protect food resources from outsiders* in order to facilitate survival. (3) *The need to protect women and children* because they represent the future survival of the tribe, and the belief that (4) *anyone who is outside the group is automatically an enemy.*

Some of these protective and exclusionary behaviors evolved from those in the lower species, where hierarchies were developed based on appearance and perceived strength, such as the *avian pecking order* phenomenon. Anthropologists argue that some of these beliefs are still deeply ingrained into the more primitive *limbic systems* of our brains, and that they may account for what we now recognize as *prejudice, racism*, and *xenophobia.* In other words, new immigration challenges the previously established social hierarchies of the inhabitants of the host country; it alters the old hierarchies and threatens the homeostasis of the group. This creates a pushback force in the form of anti-immigrant sentiment that may ultimately organize into anti-immigrant movements. The fear of loss of traditional privileges and economic loss by the dominant members of the original group plays an important role in such reactions.

Yet, humans have always evolved in the direction of adaptation and survival, and factors such as ready and rapid travel, immediate and more efficient forms of communication, better access to information and education, and transnational migration have created rapid changes in most parts of the world, leading to what has been conceptualized as the phenomenon of *globalization*. This rapid global dissemination of cultural norms, values, and beliefs across national borders facilitates individuals adopting multiple ethnic and cultural identifications in a process we can term *interculturation*, in which both the new arrivals and members of the host culture are influenced and transformed by their interactions with one another. Children, adolescents and young adults are at the forefront of such new multicultural identity formation. One of the most distinctive features of the American identity is the story of how immigrants have been absorbed into American society and how immigrants have enlarged and transformed America and the cultural identities of its inhabitants. We hope that this book will help to present a window into the future challenges that await us as a nation.

ABOUT THE AUTHORS

Eugenio M. Rothe, M.D., is Professor of Psychiatry, Founding Faculty Member of the Herbert Wertheim College of Medicine, Courtesy Professor of the Robert Stempel School of Public Health, and Adjunct Professor of the Cuban Research Institute and Latin American and Caribbean Center at Florida International University. He is a Distinguished Fellow of the American Psychiatric Association and the American Academy of Child and Adolescent Psychiatry, and a Psychoanalytic Fellow of the American Academy of Psychoanalysis and Dynamic Psychiatry. He is also board certified in Forensic Psychiatry. Dr. Rothe has dedicated his career to treating the multicultural adults, children, and families of South Florida. He has written extensively about the mental health issues of immigrants, refugees, and patients of diverse cultural backgrounds, and about psychological trauma in these populations. Dr. Rothe has been selected for the Best Doctors in America list for the past six years and is a reviewer for five scientific journals. He is President of the American Association of Social Psychiatry and the South Florida Council of Child and Adolescent Psychiatry, and Past Chair of the American Psychiatric Association's Committee for Mental Health in the Schools and the Scientific Program Committee of the American Academy of Psychoanalysis and Dynamic Psychiatry, among others. He has been the recipient of: (1) the Edward D. Harris Medical Professionalism Award of the Alpha Omega Alpha Honor Medical Society, (2) the Bruno Lima Award and (3) Nancy Roeske

Award of the American Psychiatric Association, (4) the Jeanne Spurlock Award and (5) the Distinguished Member Award of the American Academy of Child and Adolescent Psychiatry, (6) the Citation for Civilian Merit from the U.S. Armed Forces, and (7) a five-time recipient of Outstanding Teacher in Psychiatry awards from the University of Miami.

Andres J. Pumariega, M.D., is Professor and Chief of the Division of Child and Adolescent Psychiatry in the Department of Psychiatry at University of Florida College of Medicine and UF Health. He is a Distinguished Life Fellow of the American Psychiatric Association (APA) and the Academy of Child and Adolescent Psychiatry (AACAP), and Fellow of the American College of Psychiatrists and American Orthopsychiatric Association. He has served as Associate Editor of the *American Journal of Orthopsychiatry* and the *Journal of Child and Family Studies*, and on the Editorial Board of *Community Mental Health Journal* and *Journal of Child and Family Studies*, and is currently the Associate Editor of *Adolescent Psychiatry*. He co-led the drafting of the *CMHS Cultural Competence Standards* (1999) and the *AACAP Practice Parameter for Culturally Competent Child and Adolescent Psychiatric Care* (2013), the only cultural competence practice parameters in Medicine. He served as President of the American Orthopsychiatric Association (2010–2012) and President of the American Association of Social Psychiatry (2013–2015). He was the founding Chair, Work Group on Systems of Care (1994–2001), and Co-Chair, Committee on Diversity and Culture (2007–2015) in the AACAP; and Chair, Committee on Hispanic Psychiatrists (2006–2009) of the APA. He has over 220 scientific publications, published over 250 abstracts, and edited three textbooks and four journal special issues. Dr. Pumariega has received numerous awards, including the APA's *Simon Bolivar Award and Lecture in Hispanic Psychiatry* (2004) and the AACAP's *Jeanne Spurlock Award and Lecture on Diversity and Culture* (2007).

1

Culture, Identity, and Psycho-social Development

CULTURE AND IDENTITY

Culture has been defined as a socially transmitted system of ideas that (1) shapes behavior; (2) categorizes perceptions; (3) gives names to selected aspects of experience; (4) is widely shared by members of a particular society or social group; (5) functions as an orientational framework to coordinate and sanction behavior; and (6) conveys values across the generations. The *cultural process* refers to the fluid and ever-changing characteristics of a culture that respond to changes in the historical and cultural contexts in which cultures are imbedded (C. C. Hughes, 1993).

C. C. Hughes (1992) explained that it is more accurate to refer to a particular group's cultural process, which implies that a group's cultural characteristics are always evolving, rather than a group's culture, which implies that the culture is stationary. In this chapter, we use the term *culture*, although what is implied is *cultural process*. Today, we recognize that cultural values and beliefs are transmitted primarily by the family to the developing child and later reinforced by other social institutions, such as schools and other religious and community organizations. We also recognize that there are inherent biological components that contribute to the child's understanding of differences among people.

CULTURE: DEVELOPMENTAL CONSIDERATIONS

Porter (1971) noted that from the age of 3 to 4 years old, children are already capable of detecting differences in language use, and between 4 and 8 years of age, children develop a sense of ethnic identity. They identify as members of a particular ethnic group, they consolidate a sense of group identity, and they develop curiosity about other groups that are different from their own. So, cultural influences are closely related to identity formation. Cultural influences are now widely recognized as having a major impact on psychological, emotional, and even cognitive development. This impact and the diversity of developmental patterns across cultures has been recognized by cultural anthropologists as having ultimate adaptive value for humans, allowing them to overcome challenges in more diverse environments and circumstances more rapidly than natural biologic evolution would have allowed.

Starting with the birth of the child, cultures set out different expectations around parenting and childrearing and different expectations of developmental progression for children at their different stages. Cultural differences among groups have been noted by researchers around such issues as (1) the child's developmental milestones; (2) attachment; (3) maternal responsiveness; (4) children's play; (5) children's emotional reactions and expression; (6) learning and preparing for social/occupational roles; and (7) the development of a particular cultural identity (Pumariega & Joshi, 2010). For example, in a study comparing Puerto Rican, European American, and West Indian Caribbean mothers, Puerto Rican mothers expected their children to attain most milestones later. In contrast, European American mothers expected children to take first steps and become toilet trained at a later age (Pachter & Dworkin, 1997).

Cultural differences among groups have also been noted in terms of the degree of emotional attachment and emotional intensity toward one parent versus multiple caretakers or attachment to transitional objects (Winnicott, 1953) and hatching and separation–individuation (Mahler, 1974). In a study of 2,000 mother–infant pairs subjected to the *strange situation test* in eight different countries, significant cultural differences were found among the groups (Van Ijzendoorn & Kroonenberg, 1988). The degree of maternal responsiveness, including eye contact, vocalizations, and activity, also demonstrated cultural variations in a study that compared mother-infant dyads from Tokyo, Paris and New York (Bornstein et al., 1992). A study comparing Korean and Anglo-American children found cultural differences in children's social interaction, play complexity, adult–child interaction and home versus preschool play, adult beliefs about play, and children's social functioning with peers. The results suggest that children's social interaction and pretend play behavior are influenced by culture-specific socialization practices that serve adaptive functions (Farver, Kim, & Lee, 2008).

A study involving elementary school children's emotional reactions and their beliefs about revealing emotions found that Nepali-Tamang children were more likely to appraise difficult emotional situations in terms of shame, while Indian-Brahman and American-born children were more likely to endorse anger. Indian-Brahman children, in turn, were less likely to openly communicate negative emotions than the other two groups (Cole, Bruschi, & Tamang, 2003). Identity formation during adolescence and learning and preparing for social and occupational roles, which involves an interaction between self-evaluation and the internalization of values dictated by the group, represent a challenge for ethnic minorities because the adolescent sometimes has to negotiate the (1) cultural differences between their own group and the dominant group and (2) the lower or disparaged status of their group in society (Phinney, 1990).

Theorists have postulated that the development of a bicultural identity is the most adaptive resolution for ethnic identity, wherein individuals are rooted in their own culture but can selectively adopt traits of both traditional and host cultures. These issues are explored in Chapter 4, which addresses acculturation.

CULTURE AND DEVELOPMENT: OTHER EMPIRICAL FINDINGS

Significant cross-cultural research is also emerging in the areas of (1) theory of mind, (2) neural mapping, (3) object representation, and (4) emotional reactivity. *Theory of mind* is the mental representation of concepts and activities that enable humans to posit the mental states of others. Cultural variations in self-representations were found among more individualistic Westerners versus collectivists in Asian cultures, and these were found to affect emotional and cognitive processes. They can also be verified by changes seen through neuroimaging technology (Markus & Kitayama, 1991). This *cultural mapping* of brain functioning has shown differences using functional magnetic resonance imaging (fMRI) in members of collectivist versus individualistic cultures as well as differences of these two groups when compared to bicultural individuals (Chiao et al., 2009; Zhu, Zhang, Fan, & Han, 2007). These findings illustrate the dynamic influence of culture on neural representations underlying the self and, more broadly, suggest a neurobiological basis through which people acculturate, and that bicultural adaptation is cognitively based and neurally represented (Pumariega & Joshi, 2010). Neuroimaging findings also differed when observing neural processing in bilinguals versus learners of a second language, with bilinguals having distinct patterns of neural activation compared with monolinguals (Kovelman, Shalinsky, Berens, & Petitto, 2008). Another study found that adult Koreans (who do not recall their native Korean language) adopted as young children by French families and children who were French natives had similar patterns of activation to sentences spoken in French, Korean, or other foreign languages (Pallier et al., 2003).

Some studies that have involved neural responses to fear recognition by measuring greater amygdalar activation suggested that cultural exposure can affect neural processes for emotional expressions. For example, Moriguchi et al. (2005), utilizing pictures of faces of Japanese subjects, found differences in activation to fear expressions in emotion-related areas of the brain of Caucasians who had never lived in Japan compared with those of Caucasians who had lived in Japan for more than a year, suggesting that cultural exposure can affect neural processes for emotional expressions.

Prejudice has been shown to be common across cultures, time, languages, and national boundaries (Brown, 1995), and research has supported the hypothesis that prejudice is an affective state and therefore has a motivational force, usually to discharge tension or anxiety (Brehm, 1999). Prejudice is associated with stereotypes, which are beliefs and categories that are readily available and established in children's minds in early childhood before they are taught to critically evaluate perceptions (Devine, 1989). In addition, some recent research also suggested that children are prone to categorization bias, and these biases may appear as early as 3 months of age, and this early developmental propensity makes children highly susceptible to implicit stereotypical prejudices and rejection of the "other" (Bar-Haim, Ziv, Lamy, & Hodes, 2006).

A HISTORICAL PERSPECTIVE OF CULTURE AND IDENTITY FORMATION

Many of the earlier developmental theories tended to emphasize the commonalities and invariance of identity development across cultures, while more recent theories and empirical evidence tends to support a much more complex interaction between culture and child development. Freud (1856–1939) argued that the stages of feeding, toilet training, expression of sexual and competitive urges, and the achievement of intimacy in relationships were invariant across cultures; they were supposed to follow a strict chronological order, and disruptions in this order would lead to psychological problems later in life. He characterized emotions as primarily irrational and culture as providing symbolic means to assist the individual in recognizing or attenuating their impact.

In contrast, Russian psychologist Lev Semyonovich Vigotsky (1896–1934) proposed a theory of the development of *higher psychological functions* that saw human psychological development as emerging through interpersonal connections and actions with the social environment. He believed that individual mental processes had their origins in social interaction, and that identity was not a static inflexible structure of the self, but a dynamic structure that changed with the influences of the moment of human activity, its purpose, and the context and cultural characteristics of the situation.

Maria Montessori (1870–1952) viewed the first 6 years of life as essential for laying the groundwork for the internalization of positive religious, cultural, and ethical values and empathic behavior patterns. She viewed social and cognitive development as the learning and preparation that would allow children to live as members of a culture and society. She conceptualized the ages of 12 to 18 as the stage when children developed social and occupational roles that would allow them to serve not only themselves and the members of their societies but also humanity and to be able to learn how to understand the diverse viewpoints and the larger ethical dilemmas of the human condition.

Albert Bandura (1925–) has theorized that humans differ from lower animals because they are able to shape their environment, not merely be shaped by it. His concept of *human agency* distinguishes three ways in which humans shape their environment: *personal agency*, oriented toward self-regulation; *proxy agency*, through which people influence others to act on their behalf; and *collective agency*, through which people work in concert to shape their environment and their future. Bandura addressed the cultural issues of *individualism versus collectivism* and explained how the cross-cultural variations in value systems, beliefs, roles, and behaviors are variations in patterns of agency accumulated over time and reinforced by the culture and society.

The anthropologist Margaret Mead (1901–1978) was a pioneer in this research, focusing mainly on male and female gender roles, child development, and temperament and how these differed in varied cultural contexts. Mead concluded that adolescent rebellion and difficulties in adolescent transition are universal developmental givens, but that they differ significantly between cultures. She sought to explain the relationship between childrearing customs and human behaviors and saw the individual as a product of cultural values and beliefs, which shaped the person in unique ways. These cultural characteristics are learned by the individual from infancy and are reinterpreted and reinforced as the individual proceeds through subsequent developmental stages. She proposed that differences in norms and behaviors among people across different cultures are imparted from childhood, with the interaction between individuals and culture being a dynamic and complex process that results in individuals learning how to function within their society.

Vygotsky, Montessori, Mead, and Erikson, who are discussed in the next section, brought a greater awareness and depth of knowledge about the importance of culture in influencing patterns of human development, behavior, and identity formation and adaptation. They also described the adverse impact that cultural dissonance or conflict could have on the mental health of children and youth. These studies have been particularly relevant to adolescent development, in which the study of racial and ethnic identity development and the effects of acculturation have shed light on the impact on the mental health of this age group and its later manifestations in adult life (Pumariega & Joshi, 2010).

ERIKSON'S CONTRIBUTIONS TO THE UNDERSTANDING OF IDENTITY AND CULTURE

Identity formation has been historically viewed as one of the principal tasks of the passage into adulthood. Erik Erikson (1902–1994) viewed the concept of *identity* as composed of individual and social components and being closely related to the culture. He conceptualized identity as resulting from the dynamic interplay between the individual and his or her group and cultural context. Erikson (1968) added that identity development is the central task of adolescence, which culminates with the individual being able to (1) experience a subjective sense of comfort with the self; (2) having a sense of direction in life and a continuity of the self from the past, to the present, and to the anticipated future; and (3) expressing an identity that is affirmed by a community of important others (Erikson, 1959).

Erikson described how a key problem for individuals in the process of identity formation was the degree to which their own cultural identity is nurtured by members of their own culture and how it is validated by others in the community, in many ways foreseeing the dilemmas faced by youth from diverse cultural backgrounds living in host cultures (Pumariega & Joshi, 2010; Rothe, Pumariega, & Sabagh, 2011). However, this concept of the universality of development, representative of the *modernist European tradition* has been vigorously challenged. It has been considered to be based on male-oriented and Western values that are more descriptive of the White mainstream majority in the United States. The critics of this model postulate that it may not adequately represent the experiences of members of minority groups, such as adolescents born to immigrant families.

In contrast, the *postmodernist tradition* argues that identity formation is idiosyncratic, and that it is different each time and particular to every individual. In their review of the literature, Schwartz and Montgomery (2002) were unable to find any empirical studies supporting the *postmodernist tradition*; instead, their research supports a third alternative hypothesis, which argues that the fundamental structure of identity is quite consistent, but it is also influenced by variables that are particular to the individual and take into account the different styles of acculturation.

Taking this third model into account, Schwartz, Montgomery, and Briones (2006) defined identity as "the organization of self-understandings that define one's place in the world" (p. 5). They concluded that identity is a synthesis of personal, social, and cultural self-conceptions. They divided identity into (1) *personal identity*, which refers to the goals, values, and beliefs that the individual adopts and holds; (2) *social identity*, which refers to the interaction between the personal identity and the group with which one identifies; and (3) *cultural identity*, which refers to the sense of solidarity with the ideas, attitudes, beliefs, and behaviors of the members of one's ethnicity. Ethnic identity is contained within the broader concept of cultural identity, which refers to specific values, ideals, and beliefs belonging to the particular cultural group. Ethnic identity has always been a socially constructed product that is affected by a number of variables. It can recede into the background, or it can become an engulfing concern (Rothe et al., 2011), as exemplified in the case that follows.

Case I

Edgardo, a 16-year-old, brown skinned adolescent of mixed, Afro-Caribbean, Native Meso-American, and Spanish ancestry was raised by his paternal grandmother in Panama since he was 5 years old. His mother had immigrated to a small town in northern Florida, where she had progressed from being a cleaning lady to a midlevel supervisory position at the local branch of a department store chain. His mother believed that Edgardo would have better educational opportunities and the possibility of a better future in the United States and sent for him when he was 15 years old. On his arrival, Edgardo began to feel discriminated against and marginalized due to his skin color. He was cruelly teased in school by the Caucasian adolescents who did not accept him, yet he felt he had little in common with the members of the only minority group in the school, the African American adolescents, many of whom came from the small town's impoverished ghetto. Edgardo's mother was busy at work, and he had no other family members available who could offer guidance or support. He became progressively isolated and profoundly depressed; that first summer, while attending camp, he attempted to hang himself with a rope. He was hospitalized, and his mother decided to move to Miami, a multicultural and multiethnic city, where they had extended family and where Edgardo began treatment a few months

> later. He told his therapist: "In Panama I had never given any thought to my skin color since most people there are mixed, like me. I will never forget the first week I arrived in North Florida and went to the mall. I was very excited to see so many beautiful things. I walked into a clothing store, and I felt that everyone in the store was staring at me, as if I was some kind of criminal that wanted to steal something. I was very scared, and my legs began to tremble, and I turned around, left, and went home. At home I looked at myself in the mirror, began to cry, and for the first time I told myself: 'Edgardo, in this country you are not White.' I was very sad, scared, and confused.' "

This case illustrates how identity functions as a regulatory social–psychological structure and is particularly pertinent to immigrant people, who are trying to locate themselves between the culture of origin and the host culture and who are trying to maintain a sense of self-consistency while considering new possibilities (Schwartz et al., 2006).

IDENTITY AND ETHNIC–RACIAL SOCIALIZATION MESSAGES

Increased interest in racial–ethnic socialization has been precipitated by a series of complex factors, including the change in demographics that has been called the "Browning of America," in which it is expected that by the year 2035 children of color will constitute 50% of the U.S. school population. A number of recent empirical studies have documented a subtle and insidious bias against youth of color, generating negative consequences for their mental health (D. Hughes et al., 2006). The terms *racial socialization* and *ethnic socialization* refer broadly to the way that adults transmit to children information about race and ethnicity, respectively. In much of the literature, both terms overlap considerably, and the existing literature defining these terms separately is fragmented and difficult to integrate. The term *racial socialization* is mostly used to refer to studies with African Americans and in the emerging literature, but combining the terms into *ethnic–racial socialization* has served clarify the concept and prevent confusion.

Research in this area originated from the experiences of Latino, Asian, and Afro-American and Afro-Caribbean children who were facing issues of cultural retention (conserving fragments of the culture of their families), identity achievement, and in-group affiliation in the face of competing pressures to assimilate to the dominant society. Studies have consistently highlighted the fact that cultural socialization is a salient aspect of childrearing. Experiences of ethnic and racial discrimination pose a significant threat to the development and well-being of racial and ethnic minority children, but not all youth who experience discrimination are susceptible to its harmful effects, so it is important to determine which risk factors and protective factors may influence these outcomes.

A new literature has emerged describing the experience of Caribbean Blacks as they encounter American society. The ethnic–racial socialization messages given by the parents of these children may serve as a buffer against perceived discrimination and plays an important role in identity development for these second-generation Afro-Caribbean adolescents. For example, in countries of origin where Blacks are a majority, these families had a *dominant ethnic conceptualization of group membership*, and they tended to minimize racism and did not see their minority status as an impediment for social mobility (Bobb & Clarke, 2001). The opposite occurred with Black immigrants from countries where Blacks were a minority. These immigrants tended to identify with a concept of being an oppressed minority as a definition of group status (Joseph & Hunter, 2011).

These messages given by parents to their children can be categorized in four types: (1) *cultural socialization messages*, which occur at home and inform the child about the family's culture, and ethnic heritage and traditions and can promote pride or shame in one's heritage; (2) *preparation for bias messages*, which can be deliberate or implicit and inform the child about potential discrimination and provide strategies to deal with these situations; (3) *promotion of distrust messages*, which serve to encourage mistrust in *out-group members*; and (4) *mainstream socialization messages*, which encourage socialization and adoption of a mainstream identity (D. Hughes et al., 2006).

These messages vary according to the multiple variables that are encountered by the particular immigrant group. For example, Afro-Caribbeans of English colonial heritage may be more interested in fitting in, while Haitians sometimes encounter *double marginality*, discriminated by the majority culture and also stigmatized by other in-group American Blacks for being poor, of a different and unfamiliar culture, and for speaking a different language (D. Hughes et al., 2006) Paradoxically, Haitian parents transmit pride in their ethnic group to their children for their heritage of having been the first independent Black republic in the world and for their unique culture and language (Joseph & Hunter, 2011).

BIRACIAL IDENTITIES

Adolescence may be experienced as a stressful time for many youth in Western cultures because it involves establishing a unique identity while also navigating peer group norms and societal expectations. Multiracial adolescents may face a more difficult challenge than their monoracial peers in that they must develop this new identity and decide how, or even if, they can reflect positive aspects of all heritages while simultaneously rejecting certain societal expectations and stereotypes (Pumariega & Joshi, 2010). A multiracial or multiethnic heritage can further complicate this process. By adolescence, most multiracial children have been made aware of any racial–ethnic differences between classmates and themselves. Often, they are reminded of these differences as they attend school and are asked isolating questions such as, "What are you?" by classmates puzzled or threatened by their racially or ethnically mixed appearance. These alienating questions often contribute to the feeling that no one understands them, not even their monoracial parents (Kerwin & Ponterotto, 1995; Root, 1990; Wehrly, Kenney, & Kenney, 1999).

Concerns about "not fitting in" are magnified if multiracial adolescents discover that they are no longer welcome in certain peer groups because of racial issues (Diller, 1999). Additionally, some peers, and even their own parents, may pressure the adolescent to identify with only one ethnic background (Cauce et al., 1992), prompting feelings of guilt or disloyalty (Wehrly et al., 1999). Biracial youth often find themselves in a bind where they can adopt the label that society gives them; choose to identify with both racial groups or only one of those groups; or choose to be known as multiethnic (or perhaps choose another racial group altogether) (Northrup & Bean, 2007; Root, 1990). The therapist should stress that the decision is the youth's alone, and that parents should be consulted but cannot make this decision for the child. Also, they should stress that the decision need not be made immediately and that it is acceptable to change one's mind later.

Case II

Wanda was a 15-year-old girl adolescent girl of Afro-Caribbean and Puerto Rican ancestry who was born and raised in the working-class New York City neighborhood of Washington Heights. Thanks to the efforts and sacrifices of Wanda's parents and to their upward financial mobility, the family had relocated to Miami. They were residing in a neighborhood that served as an entry point into the middle class to many Hispanic immigrants in the city. Most of the inhabitants of the neighborhood were White Cubans, and Spanish and English were spoken interchangeably. Wanda spoke very little Spanish, and her coarse inner-city style clashed with her new surroundings. Wanda began arriving to school provocatively dressed and with abundant makeup, behaving in a seductive manner, charged with sexual innuendos, which captured the undivided attention of her male peers and created great commotion in the classroom. It also generated the disapproval and rejection of her female peers, who referred to her by using derogatory adjectives alluding to sexual promiscuity. The school psychologist and the consulting psychiatrist met with the school's assistant principal, who described Wanda as a "vamp," referring to a type of woman who employs sexual charms to prey on and to take advantage of men. The assistant principal insisted that, "We need to get to the bottom of this as soon as possible and try to fix the situation or this girl has to go because we cannot allow this type of 'vampish' behavior to take place in the school." On interviewing Wanda, the psychiatrist realized that she was very angry and depressed. She explained that she had been very happy living in New York, that she had never been consulted by her parents on their decision to move to Miami, and that the sudden uprooting had taken her by surprise. She said that she missed her friends and extended family in New York and admitted that she had trouble fitting in and felt out of sorts in Miami. She confessed with sadness that, "In New York I always thought of myself as Hispanic and Puerto Rican, but here the Cuban girls don't accept me because I'm too dark." The psychiatrist noticed that her accent, mannerisms, and body language appeared to be an exaggerated attempt to identify with Black inner-city youth and culture in a desperate attempt to find an ethnic group that would accept her and validate her ethnic identity. In order to help her, Wanda received individual and family therapy and antidepressant medication, and she was encouraged to write an essay about her family. In it, she described how her ancestors had been taken from Africa as slaves to the island of Puerto Rico. There, over the course of several generations, they had recovered their freedom and dignity, and shortly before Wanda's birth, her parents had immigrated to New York seeking a better future. They succeeded and eventually moved to a middle-class neighborhood in Miami. Her writing project served to highlight her family's resiliency, character, and ambition. The essay also served to validate Wanda's African, Hispanic, and American identities in a positive light.

Many teenagers will change peer groups during the course of a junior high or high school career. Frequently, when racially mixed schools are examined for the degree of integration that actually occurs, it may be surprising to learn that self-segregation with racially and ethnically similar teens is more the rule than the exception (Bronson & Merriman, 2009). In a study of approximately 750 mostly third and fourth graders in nine elementary schools in Illinois, African American children who self-segregated were more popular than African Americans who had Caucasian friends. For White children, in contrast, self-segregating seemed to hurt their popularity. "Twenty or thirty years ago Black children would not have been the ones setting the social standards, yet in this study the opposite was found to be true" (Rodkin, Wilson, & Ahn, 2007).

In the case of children and families with biracial identities, a comprehensive review of parenting practices revealed that there are three main principles that can lead to the most culturally effective parenting (Vonk, 2001); these include the following:

1. *Multicultural or racial awareness*: Knowledge of how the variables of race, ethnicity culture, language, and related power status operate in one's own and other's lives (Greene et al., 1998), including an understanding of the dynamics of racism, oppression, and other forms of discrimination (McPhatter, 1997).
2. *Multicultural planning*: Active pursuit of opportunities for transracially adopted children to learn about and participate in their culture of birth. Although socialization in the culture of one's racial group is generally congruent with the racial makeup of the family, this is not the case in families formed through transracial adoption. Furthermore, if the family is involved in other groups, such as neighborhoods, schools, and churches that are exclusively or primarily made up of European Americans, the child has no access to others of his or her birth culture. This dynamic seems to make it difficult for some adoptees to identify with, and to develop pride in, their race, ethnicity, or culture of birth (Vonk, 2001).
3. *Survival skills*: The recognition of the need for parents to prepare their children to cope successfully with racism. This skill is as important for transracial adoptees as for children

with same-race parents but may be more difficult to learn from European American parents who have had little experience of racism directed toward them. Minimizing or ignoring racial incidents is insufficient for children who may find themselves at the receiving end of racially based prejudice or discrimination. These children need help to develop strong self-images despite racism (Vonk, 2001).

LANGUAGE AND THE AMERICAN IDENTITY

Acquisition of unaccented English language has been, and continues to be, the litmus test of citizenship in the United States. In no other country are languages extinguished with such speed (Portes & Schlauffer, 1996). For immigrants, the switch to English is both an empirical fact and a cultural requirement demanded of those who have sought a new life in America. To speak *English only* is a prerequisite for social acceptance and integration, and those who try to educate their children in their mother tongue confront immense pressure for social conformity from peers, teachers, and the media. Portes and Rumbaut (1997) explained that, "In a country lacking centuries old traditions, and simultaneously receiving thousands of foreigners from the most diverse lands, language homogeneity has been seen as the bedrock of nationhood" (p. 96). Kataoka, Rowan, and Hoagwood (2009) found that in California, students with lower English language proficiency had a disproportionate impairment in difficulties with grades. Outside the ethnic enclaves that exist in the United States, to speak English only is a prerequisite for social acceptance and integration, and those who try to educate their children in their mother tongue confront immense pressure for social conformity from peers, teachers, and the media.

A number of empirical studies highlight the fact that the *first generation* learns enough English to survive economically; the *second generation* (born in the United States to immigrant parents) may use the parental tongue at home, but uses English in school; and in the *third generation*, the home language and mother tongue shift to English (Portes & Schlauffer, 1996). Language use can also have subtle connotations in everyday life in America. Waters (1996) studied first- and second-generation Blacks in New York City and noted that middle-class Blacks conveyed, through the use of mainstream English and verbal and nonverbal cues that they were not from the ghetto and that they disapproved of ghetto-specific behavior.

Case III

> Winsome, an attractive 17-year-old Afro-Caribbean girl from Barbados, had recently moved from Atlanta to Miami with her parents, who were both physicians who had recently completed their specialization training in that city. She was referred by a colleague in Atlanta in order to continue her treatment for attention deficit disorder–inattentive type. Winsome shared in therapy that, "I feel much better here in Miami, and I am also doing better in school. There are more people from the islands here, so I don't have to keep explaining where I'm from. In Atlanta, the Black kids in school said that I 'talked funny' and were always telling me that I was trying to 'act white' because I wasn't getting into trouble and because sometimes I dated white kids. Here I can be myself and talk like myself, and people have even said they think my accent is 'cool.' "

This case is an example of how speaking "accented English," even by a native English speaker, can serve to highlight socioeconomic and cultural differences that can separate the adolescent from particular peer groups. This example also helps to validate how immigrating to a more pluralistic urban area, where there is an ethnic enclave of compatriots, facilitates acculturation and operates as a protective factor for mental health outcomes. Language retention is closely related to socioeconomic variables. For example, immigrant children growing up in impoverished communities receive no encouragement to retain their parent's native language because the native language is stigmatized as a symbol of lower status (Portes &

Schlauffer, 1996). This is very much the case of second-generation Haitian youth of working-class parents in Miami, who rapidly shed Haitian Creole for English and prefer to be identified as American rather than Haitian American.

In contrast, Portes and Stepic (1993) studied language utilization in Miami, Florida. They found that Spanish was "alive and well" among first-generation Cuban immigrants, but that language retention decreased in proportion to the length of stay in the United States. They found that, in spite of the economic prosperity, excellent self-esteem, and social support offered by the Cuban "ethnic enclave" in Miami, 90% of second-generation Cubans preferred to communicate in English.

The interplay between the immigrant parents and their children in the second generation also accounts for the type of *goodness of fit* (Winnicott, 1988) that will occur in the acculturation process into the United States. *Generational consonance* occurs when parents and children acculturate at the same rate or when the parents encourage selective acculturation among the second generation, such that the cultural harmony between parents and children is maintained while allowing the children to effectively adapt to the new American reality. *Cultural dissonance* occurs when the second generation is neither guided nor accompanied by the changes in the first generation. *Consonant resistance* to acculturation occurs among isolated immigrant groups that are strongly oriented toward returning to their country of origin and their presence in the host society has been temporary, such as in the case of exiles (Portes & Rumbaut, 1997; Rothe et al., 2011).

IDENTITY, PSYCHO-SOCIAL FUNCTIONING, AND RESILIENCE

Schwartz, Zamboanga, Weisskirch, and Wang (2009) examined the relationship between personal and cultural identity and risk factors among emerging adults. They found that confusion emerged as a negative predictor of self-esteem and optimism and as a positive predictor of depressive symptoms, rule breaking, unprotected sex, and cigarette use.

Identity *coherence*, on the other hand, positively predicted optimism and negatively predicted rule breaking and aggression. However, these investigators also found that *personal identity* related to well-being and internalizing symptoms more strongly than *cultural identity*, and that it is imperative not to lose sight of the emerging adult's core identity development. These findings seem to indicate that an understanding of "who one is and where one is going" is more critical than understanding where one fits within one's ethnic group and the context where one resides. Despite the fact that cultural identity was a significant mediator and that cultural identity influences personal identity in implicit or indirect ways, targeting personal identity directly may serve as the most optimal mechanism for promoting both cultural identity and positive psycho-social functioning.

In an influential article examining the cultural aspects of resilience, Cameron, Ungar, and Liebenberg (2007) described the "scaffolding" that characterizes successful adaptation to adversity across cultures, which includes familial, environmental, cultural, social, psychological, and physiologic processes. Using an attachment paradigm, the authors cited international data (Ungar, Lee, Callaghan, & Boothroyd, 2005; Ungar & Liebenberg, 2005) supporting the idea that "children [and youth] seen by their communities as resilient demonstrate complexity in how they negotiate relational resources to protect themselves against personal and environmental stressors" (Cameron et al., 2007, p. 296). The authors identified seven *tensions* requiring resolution to achieve healthy psycho-social development by the end of adolescence (Cameron et al., 2007, pp. 296–297).

1. *Access to material resources*: The availability of structural provisions, including financial assistance and education, and the provision of basic instrumental needs such as food, shelter, clothing, access to medical care, and employment, which are a function of the security of family, peer, and community relationships. Although primary caregivers are key to ensuring availability, they are not able to provide everything engaged adolescents require as their needs become more complex.

2. *Relationships:* Study participants used the matrix of their relationships to negotiate access to the resources necessary to cope with their surroundings. These relationships included networks of family members, peers, adults in their communities, teachers, mentors, role models, intimate partners, and even enemies who could be manipulated to achieve status-related goals, such as being perceived as powerful or empathetic.
3. *Identity*: A sense of individuality has to be negotiated through relationships with others. Assertions such as, "I am," "I believe." and "I feel" are ways youth validate a bounded sense of self. The process of this identity formation, however, was described as one of *coconstruction through mutual discursive spaces*.
4. *Cohesion*: In contrast to the theme of individuality, participants identified the need to balance one's sense of responsibility to self and duty to one's broader community as critical to healthy development. This construct of cohesion borrows theoretically from the social capital theory. The complexity of adolescent attachments that result from ecologic diversity demands attention to the needs of others in a reflexive process that nurtures the self.
5. *Power and control*: Attachments at multiple ecologic levels bring with them the basis for shared and self-agency experiences of power to make decisions and the control to enact them. These experiences must be found through interactions in shared relational spaces.
6. *Cultural adherence*: Adherence, or standing in opposition to cultural norms, demands complex negotiations with caregivers and communities. Culture clashes between localized family and cultural norms and global culture (often synonymous with popular culture) is a function of the relationships experienced by the youth.

7. *Social justice*: In the expanding topography of children's relationships, they develop the capacity to individually and collectively assert their rights. Experiences of prejudice and dynamics of sociopolitical disenfranchisement that often come with exposure to risk (e.g., poverty, disability, or racial prejudice) can be catalysts for building a social conscience and resistance (Pumariega & Joshi, 2010).

OTHER INFLUENCES ON DEVELOPMENT

Discussing religion and spirituality with patients is often controversial, and the mental health professional should always refrain from giving opinions or making value judgments when these topics are breached. However, according to a recent qualitative research review, most children in the United States consider themselves spiritual beings, and therefore these investigators suggested that clinicians should inquire about a child's spiritual or religious life. Furthermore, families may benefit greatly when clinicians use spiritual or religious resources as adjuncts in treatment if these are perceived as helpful for the family or child in coping better with the current situation (Houskamp, Fisher, & Stuber, 2004).

A more practical and empirically based approach of addressing religion and spirituality can be done by utilizing a brief screen to help structure questions better, with the acronym FICA: (1) The letter *F* represents the question, "Is religious faith an important part of your day-to-day or weekly life?" This question could be followed by other questions about formal religious affiliation and level of spirituality. (2) The letter *I* represents the question, "How has faith influenced your life, past and present?" This question may uncover important spiritual experiences. (3) The letter *C* represents the question, "Are you (or is your family) currently a part of a religious or spiritual community?" This question can help clarify the role a spiritual community might play in treatment interventions. (4) Finally, the letter *A* represents the question, "What are the spiritual needs that you would like me to address?" This question allows the clinician to identify spiritual areas that may become part of a treatment plan (Josephson & Wiesner, 2004; Puchalski & Romer, 2000). Another approach involves the use of two screening questions developed by Matthews et al. (1998): "Is religion or spirituality important to you (or your child-teen)?" and "What can I do to support your faith or religious commitment?"

CONCLUSIONS

A major task of emerging adulthood involves exploring and consolidating a sense of identity, so understanding who one is, at both the personal and sociocultural levels, is of critical importance for a successful transition into adulthood, especially in the face of increasing globalization and ethnic and cultural diversity. In the recent past, cultural identity had been studied in minority groups, with Whites used as a comparison, but the onset of globalization and the decreasing importance of national boundaries have rendered cultural identity important for both minority and majority group members. In previous studies, orientation toward American cultural practices among second-generation immigrants and beyond has been associated with negative psycho-social outcomes such as behavior problems, drug use, sexual risk taking, and poor nutrition. However, many of these studies used unidimensional models of cultural identity where heritage and American cultural orientations were cast as opposing ends of a continuum.

New research findings suggest that parallel lines of development for personal and cultural identity relate to psycho-social functioning through a consolidated sense of personal identity, and that personal identity, or "who one is and where one is going," is more critical than understanding where one fits within one's ethnic group and the context where one resides. So, targeting personal identity directly may serve as the most optimal mechanism for promoting both cultural identity and positive psycho-social functioning. In multicultural societies, identifying with one or both sets of cultural values and practices may contribute to helping to consolidate a sense of self in emerging adulthood. In turn, a consolidated sense of self may contribute to a positive functioning personal and cultural identity. Ultimately, contact between individuals from different ethnic and cultural backgrounds may lead to exploration (and perhaps consolidation) of both personal and cultural aspects of identity, and these constructs may also apply to immigrants and nonimmigrants beyond the second generation (Schwartz et al., 2006, 2009).

REFERENCES

Bar-Haim, Y., Ziv, T., Lamy, D., & Hodes, R. M. (2006). Nature and nurture in own-race face processing. *Psychological Science, 17*, 159–163.

Bobb, V. F. B., & Clarke, A. Y. (2001). Experiencing success: Structuring the perception of opportunities for West Indians. In N. Foner (Ed.), *Islands in the city: West Indian migration to New York* (pp. 216–236). Los Angeles: University of California Press.

Bornstein, M., Tamis-LeMonda, C., Tal, J., et al. (1992). Maternal responsiveness to infants in three societies: The United States, France, and Japan. *Child Development. 63*, 808–821.

Brehm, J. (1999). The intensity of emotion. *Personality and Social Psychology Review, 3*, 2–22.

Bronson, P., & Merriman, A. (2009). *Nurture shock*. New York: Hachette Book Group.

Brown, R. (1995). *Prejudice: Its social psychology*. London: Blackwell.

Cameron, C. A., Ungar, M., & Liebenberg, L. (2007). Cultural understandings of resilience: roots for wings in the development of affective resources for resilience. *Child and Adolescent Psychiatric Clinics of North America, 16*, 285–301.

Cauce, A. M., Hiraga, Y., Mason, C., Aguilar, T., Ordonez, N., & Gonzales, N. (1992). Between a rock and a hard place: Social adjustment of biracial youth. In: M. P. Root (Ed.), *Racially mixed people in America* (pp. 207–222). Newbury Park, CA: Sage.

Chiao, J., Harada, T., Komeda, H., et al. (2009). Dynamic cultural influences on neural representations of the self. *Journal of Cognitive Neuroscience, 22*, 1–11.

Cole, P., Bruschi, C., & Tamang, B. (2003). Cultural differences in children's emotional reactions to difficult situations. *Child Development, 73*, 983–996.

Devine, P. (1989). Stereotypes and prejudice: Their automatic and controlled components. *Journal of Personality and Social Psychology, 44*, 20–33.

Diller, J. V. (1999). *Cultural diversity: A primer for the human services*. Toronto: Wadsworth.

Erikson, E. (1959). *Childhood and society*. New York: Norton.

Erikson, E. (1968). *Identity, youth, and crisis*, New York: Norton.

Farver, J., Kim, Y., & Lee, Y. (2008). Cultural differences in Korean- and Anglo-American preschoolers' social interaction and play behaviors. *Child Development, 66*, 1088–1099.

Greene, R. R., Watkins, M., McNutt, I., et al. (1998). Diversity defined. In R. R. Greene & M. Watkins (Eds.), *Serving diverse constituencies* (pp. 29–57). New York: Aldine de Gruyter.

Houskamp, B. M., Fisher, L. A., & Stuber, M. L. (2004). Spirituality in children and adolescents: Research findings and implications for clinicians and researchers. *Child and Adolescent Psychiatric Clinics of North America, 13*, 221–230.

Hughes, C. C. (1992). "Ethnography": What's in a word—Process? Product? Promise? *Qualitative Health Research, 2*, 4. 439–450.

Hughes, C. C. (1993). Culture in clinical psychiatry. In A. C. Gaw (Ed.), *Culture, ethnicity and mental illness*. Washington, DC: Psychiatric Press.

Hughes, D., Rodriguez, J., Smith, E. P., Johnson, D. J., Stevenson, H. C., & Spicer, P. (2006). Parents' ethnic-racial socialization practices: A review of research and directions for future study. *Developmental Psychology, 42*(5), 747–770.

Joseph, N., & Hunter, C. D. (2011). Ethnic-racial socialization messages in the identity development of second-generation Haitians. *Journal of Adolescent Research, 26*(3), 344–380.

Josephson, A. M., & Wiesner, I. S. (2004). Worldview in psychiatric assessment. In: A. M. Josephson & J. R. Peteet (Eds.), *Handbook of spirituality and worldview in clinical practice* (pp. 15–30). Washington, DC: American Psychiatric Press.

Kataoka, S. H., Rowan, B., & Hoagwood, K. E. (2009). Bridging the divide: In search of common ground in mental health and education research and policy. *Psychiatric Services, 6*(11), 1510–1515.

Kerwin, C., & Ponterotto, J. G. (1995). Biracial identity development: Theory and research. In J. P. Ponterotto, J. M. Casas, L. A. Suzuki, et al. (Eds.), *Handbook of multicultural counseling* (pp. 199–217). Thousand Oaks, CA: Sage.

Kovelman, I., Shalinsky, M., Berens, M., & Petitto, L. A. (2008). Shining new light on the brain's "bilingual signature": A functional near infrared spectroscopy investigation of semantic processing. *NeuroImage, 39*, 1457–1471.

Mahler, M. (1974). On the first three subphases of the separation-individuation process. *International Journal of Psychoanalysis, 3*, 295–306.

Markus, H., & Kitayama, S. (1991). Culture and the self: Implications for cognition, emotion, and motivation. *Psychological Review, 98*, 224–253.

Matthews, D. A., McCullough, M. E., Larson, D. B., Koenig, H. G., Swyers, J. P., & Milano, M. G. (1998). Religious commitment and health status: A review of the research and implications for family medicine. *Archives of Family Medicine, 7*, 118–124.

McPhatter, A. R. (1997). Cultural competence in *child welfare*: What is it? How do we achieve it? What happens without it? *Child Welfare, 76*, 255–278.

Moriguchi, Y., Ohnishi, T., Kawachi, T., et al. (2005). Specific brain activation in Japanese and Caucasian people to fearful faces. *NeuroReport, 16*, 133–136.

Northrup, J. C., & Bean, R. A. (2007). Culturally competent family therapy with Latino Anglo-American adolescents: Facilitating identity formation. *The American Journal of Family Therapy, 35*, 251–263.

Pachter, L., & Dworkin, P. (1997). Maternal expectations about normal child development in 4 cultural groups. *Archives of Pediatrics and Adolescent Medicine, 151*, 1144–1150.

Pallier, C., Dehaene, S., Poline, J., et al. (2003). Brain imaging of language plasticity in adopted adults: Can a second language replace the first? *Cerebral Cortex, 13*, 155–161.

Phinney, J. (1990). Ethnic identity in adolescents and adults: Review of research. *Psychological Bulletin, 10*, 499–514.

Porter, J. (1971). *White child–Black child: The development of racial attitudes*. Cambridge, MA: Harvard University Press.

Portes, A., & Rumbaut, R. G. (1997). *Immigrant America: A portrait.* 2nd ed. Berkeley, CA: University of California Press.

Portes, A., & Schlauffer, R. (1996). Language and the second generation bilingualism yesterday and today. In A. Portes (Ed.), *The new second generation* (pp. 197–220). New York: Russell Sage.

Portes, A., & Stepic, A. (1993). *City on the Edge: The Transformation of Miami*. Berkely, CA: University of California Press.

Puchalski, C. M., & Romer, A. L. (2000). Taking a spiritual history allows clinicians to understand patients more fully. *Journal of Palliative Medicine, 3*, 129–137.

Pumariega, A. J., & Joshi, S. (2010). Culture and development in children and youth. *Child and Adolescent Psychiatry Clinics of North America, 19*(4), 661–680.

Rodkin, P. C., Wilson, T., & Ahn, H. J. (2007). Social integration between African American and European American children in majority Black, majority White, and multicultural elementary classrooms. In P. C. Rodkin & L. D. Hanish (Eds.), *Social network analysis and children's peer relationships* (pp. 25–42). San Francisco: Jossey-Bass.

Root, M. P. (1990). Resolving "other" status: Identity development of biracial individuals. In L. S. Brown & M. P. Root (Eds.), *Diversity and complexity in feminist therapy* (pp. 185–205). New York: Haworth.

Rothe, E. M., Pumariega, A. J., & Sabagh, D. (2011). Identity and acculturation in immigrant and second generation adolescents. *Adolescent Psychiatry, 1*(1), 72–81.

Schwartz, S. J., & Montgomery, M. J. (2002). Similarities or differences in identity development? The impact of acculturation and gender on identity process and outcomes. *Journal of Youth and Adolescence, 31*, 359–372.

Schwartz, S. J., Montgomery, M. J., & Briones, E. (2006). The role of identity in acculturation among immigrant people: Theoretical propositions, empirical questions, and applied recommendations. *Human Development, 49*, 1–30.

Schwartz, S. J., Zamboanga, B. L., Weisskirch, R. S., & Wang, S. C. (2009). The relationships of personal and cultural identity to adaptive and maladaptive psychosocial functioning in emerging adults. *Journal of Social Psychology, 150*(1), 1–33.

Ungar, M., Lee, A. W., Callaghan, T., & Boothroyd, R. A. (2005). An international collaboration to study resilience in adolescents across cultures. *Journal of Social Work Research, 6*(1), 5–24.

Ungar, M., & Liebenberg, L. (2005). The International Resilience Project: A mixed methods approach to the study of resilience across cultures. In M. Ungar (Ed.), *Handbook for working with children and youth: Pathways to resilience across cultures and contexts* (pp. 211–226). Thousand Oaks, CA: Sage.

Van Ijzendoorn, M., & Kroonenberg, P. (1988). Cross-cultural patterns of attachment: A metaanalyis of the strange situation. *Child Development, 59*, 147–156.

Vonk, M. E. (2001). Cultural competence for transracial adoptive parents. *Social Work, 46*(3), 246–255.

Waters, M. C. (1996). Ethnic and racial identities of second-generation Black immigrants in New York City. In A. Portes (Ed.), *The new second generation* (pp. 177). New York: Russell Sage.

Wehrly, B., Kenney, K. R., & Kenney, M. E. (1999). *Counseling multiracial families.* Thousand Oaks, CA: Sage.

Winnicott, D. W. (1953). Transitional objects and transitional phenomena—A study of the first not-me possession. *The International Journal of Psycho-Analysis, 34,* 89–97.

Winnicott, D. W. (1988). *The maturational processes and the facilitating environment.* 11th ed. Madison, WI: International Universities Press.

Zhu, Y., Zhang, L., Fan, J., & Han, S. (2007). Neural basis of cultural influence on self-representation. *NeuroImage, m34,* 1310–1316.

2

Immigration Trends in the United States

Migration to seek economic or material improvement, or to move from a hostile and persecutory environment to a more generous and welcoming one, has been an important human activity throughout the course of history. Currently, migration to the United States occurs through legal and illegal paths. The United States accepts the highest percentage of immigrants and refugees of any nation on Earth. The total number of immigrants in the United States is estimated at 40 million, and between 2000 and 2010, the United States received 14 million immigrants, the highest decade of immigration in the nation's history. The nation's immigrant population has doubled since 1990, nearly tripled since 1980, and quadrupled since 1970, when it stood at 9.7 million. The states with the largest numerical increases over the last decade were California, Texas, Florida, New York, New Jersey, Georgia, Virginia, North Carolina, Maryland, Washington, Illinois, Pennsylvania, and Massachusetts.

Latin America contributed the most immigrants, with 58% arriving from this region from 2000 to 2010. Mexico was by far the top immigrant-sending country, accounting for 29% of all immigrants (21 million) in 2000 to 2010. The median age of immigrants in 2010 was 41.4 compared to 35.9 for natives. While the number of immigrants in the country is higher than at any time in American history, the immigrant share of the population (12.9%) was actually higher 90 years ago when a large wave of immigrants arrived from Europe. It is tempting to oversimplify and state that poverty in the country of origin and strong job markets in the receiving country are the principal reasons to emigrate.

If we take into account that there were two significant recessions between 2000 and 2001—plus the September 11 terrorist attacks, no job growth, and an overall net loss of jobs between 2000 and 2010—in spite of this immigration to the United States remained at an all-time high, with 13.9 million immigrants (legal and illegal) arriving between 2000 and 2010. This is a reminder that immigration is a complex process and not simply a function of labor market conditions in the United States. Many factors influence migration decisions, such as a desire to be with relatives, the political freedoms that are found in the United States and are present in very few countries around the world, and the generosity of American public services. Immigration is also driven, in part, by the social networks of family and friends that provide information to the future immigrant and facilitate the immigrant's adaptation once arriving in the receiving country (Camarota, 2011).

Immigrant children and the children of immigrants also comprise an increasing proportion of America's younger population. Immigrants account for over 12.9% of the U.S. population, but their children are over 23% of the population under the age of 18, and about 2.2 million children in the United States are recent immigrants. Seventy-five percent of children of immigrants were born in the United States and are thus U.S. citizens. The majority of the children of immigrants—61% in 2003—live in families where one or more children are citizens but one or more parents are noncitizens. First-generation (children who were born outside the United States but immigrated) and second-generation immigrant children (children who were born in the United States and who have one or both parents who are immigrant) are the most rapidly growing segment of the U.S. child population and account for over 30% of the U.S. school population (U.S. Census, 2014).

TYPES OF IMMIGRANTS

The circumstances that determine a person's decision to migrate may vary. The types of immigrants have been classified as follows: (1) *Financial immigrants* arrive in the United States in an attempt to improve their financial situation and provide for their families in a manner not available in their country of origin. They are searching for the proverbial American dream. (2) *Intellectual, professional, or student immigrants* arrive in the United States in a quest for knowledge, professional advancement, or educational opportunities not available to them in their country of origin. (3) *Refugees* are those who are displaced by war, persecution, or natural disasters and are resettled in the receiving countries, sometimes by agreements between international aid organizations and the countries that have agreed to receive the refugees. (4) *Asylum seekers* are those who chose to seek sanctuary in a new country because of fear of persecution or violence. (5) *Sojourners* are those who relocate to a new country on a time-limited basis and for a specific purpose, with full intentions to return to their countries of origin after that period of time is over. In this category, one finds international students or corporate executives who are sent overseas for professional reasons. Also included are migrant workers who follow the seasonal crops and are often subjected to financial abuses, with their children suffering many discontinuities in schooling. Ultimately, there are the (6) *exiles*, who have left their countries of origin by way of banishment or expulsion and are forbidden to return, leaving them to deal with complicated mourning processes. The word *exile* derives from the Greek *ex-ilia* (*Ilia*, "the city of Troy"; *ex*, "no longer"), meaning "no longer Troy." In ancient Greece, exile was considered a form of cruel and usual punishment (Grinberg & Grinberg, 1989).

THE CHANGING IMMIGRANT ETHNICITIES

Until the mid-twentieth century, the United States received predominantly European immigrants, whose racial and cultural characteristics allowed them to assimilate rapidly into the American social fabric. In the past 40 years, immigration from Europe and Canada has declined dramatically, and non-European immigration has increased. By the year 2050, European-origin Americans will no longer be the numerical majority. This has already happened among 6-year-olds and will happen before 2030 among children younger than 18 years (U.S. Census, 2014). The majority of the new immigrants to the United States describe themselves as non-White, and immigrants from the Caribbean and Central and South America are the most racially mixed, with less than 45% self-reporting as White. This rapidly changing demographic landscape in the United States, with an increasing multiracial and multicultural population, is a result of three major factors: (1) the progressive aging and low birth rate of its European-origin population; (2) the lower mean ages and increasing birth rates in non-European minority groups; and (3) a significant increase in immigration from Latin America, Asia, and Africa. Given current immigration trends and birth rates, virtually 93% of the growth of the nation's working-age population between now and 2050 will be accounted for by immigrants and their U.S.-born children. By then, the nation's "immigrant stock" (first- and second-generations combined, adults and children combined) could grow from 76 million now to more than 160 million, at which point it would comprise a record share (37%) of the U.S. population (Passel, 2006). These growing populations are diverse in their racial, ethnic, national origin, immigration, and socioeconomic makeup, and as a group, they are different from the older, European-origin, White, and higher socioeconomic mainstream population. All of these differences are discussed in more detail in other chapters of this book.

There has been much recent controversy about the entry of undocumented immigrants into the United States and of any efforts to legalize their status. This debate has contributed to an increasing anti-immigrant sentiment in a nation that paradoxically has been built by immigrants.

Nativist movements have been common in the history of immigration to the United States, and the largely non-European composition of the current immigrant population contributes to fuel these recent sentiments. Some of the arguments are cultural, including concerns that the new immigrants are not learning English and are not assimilating as did earlier European immigrants. Other arguments focus on the economic drain that undocumented immigrants may pose for states and communities, through both competition for jobs and expenditures for health and human services (Pumariega & Rothe, 2010; Rothe, Pumariega, & Sabagh, 2011).

UNAUTHORIZED IMMIGRANTS

Most of the immigrants (two thirds) who arrived in the United States in the last two decades did so by legal means, and it is estimated that there were 11.3 million illegal immigrants living in the United States by 2013 (Pew Research Center, 2013). Other estimates have reported higher numbers of unauthorized immigrants, placing these numbers between 10.9 and 15.7 million (Markon, 2016). Undocumented immigrant workers are a major source of entry-level labor in the United States (farm labor, service workers, construction workers, etc.). Such workers perform work that U.S. residents and citizens generally are not willing to do.

There are 3.6 million unauthorized immigrants who do not live with a spouse, partner, or children. These "unpartnered adults without children" are 35% of unauthorized adult immigrants; their numbers have remained unchanged since 2005. The number of children of unauthorized immigrants increased by 1.2 million from 2003 to 2008, despite the fact that the number of unauthorized immigrants under age 18 has remained roughly constant.

These findings suggest that the demographics of unauthorized immigrants is changing from one of adult males alone to one of entire families that are not legally authorized to reside in the United States. In 2003, of the 4.3 million children of unauthorized immigrants, 2.7 million, or 63%, were born in the United States. In 2008, of the 5.5 million children of unauthorized immigrants, 4 million, or 73%, were born in the United States. Due to the timing of arrival to the United States by their parents, the youngest children of unauthorized immigrants are considerably more likely than older ones to be U.S. citizens. Among children under age 6 whose parents are unauthorized immigrants, 91% were born in the United States, in contrast with those whose ages are between 14 to 17 years. Of the latter group, 50% were born in the United States. These findings point to a trend in which children of unauthorized immigrants are becoming American and integrating into the mainstream.

Most unauthorized immigrants live with a spouse or cohabiting partner (4.3 million) and also live with their children under 18. Nearly half of all adult unauthorized immigrants (48%) live with their children, and nearly all 1.5 million unauthorized immigrant children live with their parents. Mixed-status family groups (i.e., families with unauthorized immigrants and their U.S. citizen children) consist of 8.8 million people. Of these, 3.8 million are unauthorized immigrant adults, and half a million are unauthorized immigrant children. The number of people in mixed-status families has grown in concert with the increasing unauthorized immigrant population. The 8.8 million people in these families are a slight majority (53%) of the nation's 16.6 million unauthorized immigrants and their family members.

Seen from a different perspective, 3.8 million unauthorized immigrants are parents of children who are U.S. citizens, and these figures have not changed since 2003. These numbers indicate that the vast majority of all children with at least one unauthorized immigrant parent live in two-parent families (80%). This is similar to the share of children of other immigrants who do so (84%) and higher than the share of children with U.S.-born parents (71%). They also indicate that deportation of an unauthorized parent will cause severe family disruptions in the majority of these families.

In terms of their education, adult unauthorized immigrants are disproportionately likely to be poorly educated. Among 25- to 64-year-old unauthorized immigrants, 47% have less than a high school education, 29% have less than a ninth-grade education, and less than 27% have completed high school but gone no further. In contrast, 31% U.S.-born residents completed high school. Surprisingly, the percentage of high school graduates among legal immigrants is slightly lower at 24%. By contrast, only 8% of U.S.-born residents ages 25–64 have not graduated from high school. In terms of college education, among unauthorized immigrants only 25% have attended or graduated from college, compared to 54% of legal immigrants and 61% of U.S.-born residents. Arriving at a young age to the United States increases the possibilities of attaining a college education for unauthorized immigrants. Among those who arrived before age 14, 61% are in college or have attended college. However, this trend for college continuation is still considerably lower than the rate for legal immigrants (76%) or U.S.-born residents (71%).

Because unauthorized immigrants are less likely to have a formal education, they tend to be overrepresented in several sectors of the economy, including agriculture, construction, leisure/hospitality, and services. These lower levels of education also lead these undocumented immigrants to have lower household incomes. In 2007, the median household income of unauthorized immigrants was $36,000, well below the $50,000 median household income for U.S.-born residents. In contrast to other immigrants, undocumented immigrants do not attain markedly higher incomes the longer they live in the United States. Undocumented immigrants and their U.S.-born children account for 11% of people with incomes below the poverty level, which is twice the rate of poverty of the total population (5.5%). A third of the children of unauthorized immigrants and a fifth of adult unauthorized immigrants live in poverty. This is nearly double the poverty rate for children of U.S.-born parents (18%) or of U.S.-born adults (10%). In 2007, more than half of adult unauthorized immigrants (59%) and 45% of their children had no health insurance. In contrast, 25% of children born in the United States were uninsured. Because of these high proportions without health insurance, unauthorized immigrants and their children account for one in six Americans without health insurance (17%), more than three times their representation in the population.

Ironically, undocumented immigrant men aged 18–64 are more likely to be in the labor force than are men who are legal immigrants or who were born in the United States. Among men of working age, 94% of undocumented immigrants are in the labor force, compared with 85% of legal immigrant men and 83% of U.S.-born men. The opposite is true for women. Only 58% of working-age women who are undocumented immigrants are in the labor force, well below the share of women who are U.S. born (73%) or legal immigrants (66%). The major reason for this is that a higher share of women who are unauthorized immigrants are not working because they are raising children at home, 29%, compared with 16% of other immigrants and 8% of U.S.-born women.

The unauthorized immigrant share of the labor force varies greatly by state. Approximately 1 in 10 workers in Nevada, California, and Arizona is an unauthorized immigrant. Most states, however, are below average in the share of unauthorized immigrants in their labor force, with 36 states having less than 1 in 20 workers who are unauthorized immigrants (Passel, 2006).

ECONOMIC ATTAINMENT

The 20 million second-generation Americans, adult U.S.-born children of immigrants, are substantially better off than immigrants themselves on key measures of socioeconomic attainment. They have higher incomes; more are college graduates and homeowners; and fewer live in poverty. In all of these measures, their characteristics resemble those of the full U.S. adult population. Also, second-generation Hispanics and Asian Americans place more importance than does the general public on hard work and career success. They are more inclined to call themselves liberal and less likely to identify as Republicans. And, for the most part, they are more likely to say their standard of living is higher than that of their parents at the same stage of life. In all of these measures, the second generation resembles the immigrant generation more closely than the general public.

Adults in the second generation are doing better than those in the first generation in terms of their median household income ($58,000 vs.

$46,000); more of them have college degrees (36% vs. 29%); and more are homeowners (64% vs. 51%). They are less likely to be in poverty (11% vs. 18%) and less likely not to finish high school (10% vs. 28%). Most of these favorable comparisons hold up in comparison to other ethnic subgroups and with White Americans. There is a marked difference in poverty by nativity among children of legal immigrants. The poverty rate is higher for legal immigrant children born abroad (29%) than for the children of legal immigrants born in the United States (17%). For children of U.S.-born parents, 18% are in poverty, a figure not substantially different from the rate for U.S.-born children of legal immigrants. About 78% of second-generation Hispanics and 72% of Asian Americans believe that if they work hard, they can get ahead in the United States. In contrast, only 58% of the adult U.S. population feels the same way (Passel, 2006).

INTERGROUP RELATIONS, VALUES, AND POLITICAL ORIENTATION

Among the first-generation immigrants, 26% of Latinos and 49% of Asian Americans say that they get along well with the other major ethnic groups. This improves dramatically among the second generation, with 52% of Latinos and 64% of Asian Americans stating that their group gets along well with all other major racial and ethnic groups in America. The second generations of these groups are also more likely than the immigrants to say they have friends outside their ethnic group or country-of-origin group. Only 8% of immigrants and only 8% of all U.S. adults have a spouse of an ethnic or racial group different from their own. This increases slightly to 15% among the total of second-generation immigrants. However, interethnic or interracial marriage is higher among Latinos (26%) and Asians (23%).

Among Latinos and Asian Americans, both the first and the second generation identify more with the Democratic Party than with the Republican Party and characterize themselves as liberal, as opposed to conservative. Among the second generation of both groups, more than half believe that abortion should be legal and that homosexuality should be accepted by society. In what appears to be a form of reverse assimilation, 41% of second-generation women were unmarried when they gave birth, compared with 23% of first-generation immigrant women and 36% among all women in the U.S. population. This trend was highest among second-generation Latino women at 52% (Pew Research Center, 2013).

CONCLUSIONS

The United States has been the top destination for international migrants since at least 1960, with one fifth of the world's migrants living there as of 2018. Despite its long history of immigration, the United States has oscillated between perceiving immigration as a valuable resource and as a major challenge (Zong, Batalova, & Hallock, 2019). A more recent and unnoticed trend in immigration is the so-called brain gain because 48% of immigrants who arrived in the United States between 2011 and 2015 are college graduates, the great majority are bilingual, and those immigrants with temporary visas are the most educated. One in two college graduates is from Asia, particularly China, India, and the Philippines. In addition, Latin Americans are now the second-largest group of skilled immigrants following American born workers, with Europeans occupying the third place. The numbers of highly skilled immigrants have grown over the past 15 years (Batalova & Fix, 2017).

The most contentious issue in immigration today is how to stop and what to do about the more than 11 million unauthorized immigrants residing in the United States. Unauthorized immigration is made possible, in part, by a web of false documents and international smuggling networks that constitute a risk to national security. These individuals who have no legal status have minimal rights, are subjected to many forms of exploitation, and exist in a limbo that impedes progress toward immigrant integration. A comprehensive government reform of the immigration system should include agreements with countries that contribute immigrants to the United States in order to manage labor flows in the context of economic interdependence with the purpose of promoting mutual national growth and security. A comprehensive set of recommendations for immigration reform is available (Abraham et al., 2006).

In addition to these recommendations, it is important to take into account that the unauthorized immigrants who are already residing in the United States are making important economic contributions to the nation's productivity, competitiveness, and fiscal health. Providing an earned path to permanent legal status to these individuals would increase tax revenues due to the increased earning power from having legal status.

REFERENCES

Abraham, S., Hamilton, L. H., Meissner, D., Meyers, D. W., Papademetriou, D. G., & Fix, M. (2006, September). Immigration and America's future: A new chapter. Migration Policy Institute report. https://www.migrationpolicy.org/research/immigration-and-americas-future-new-chapter. Accessed December 25, 2018.

Batalova, J., & Fix, M. (2017, May). New brain gain: Rising human capital among recent immigrants to the United States. Migration Policy Institute fact sheet. https://www.migrationpolicy.org/research/new-brain-gain-rising-human-capital-among-recent-immigrants-united-states. Accessed December 25, 2018.

Camarota, S. (2011). A record-setting decade of immigration: 2000–2010. Center for Immigration Studies. https://cis.org/Report/RecordSetting-Decade-Immigration-20002010. Accessed December 15, 2018.

Grinberg, L., & Grinberg, R. (1989). *Psychoanalytic perspectives on migration and exile*. New Haven, CT: Yale University Press.

Markon, J. (2016, January 20). U.S. illegal immigrant population falls below 11 million, continuing nearly decade-long decline, report says. *The Washington Post*. https://www.washingtonpost.com/news/federal-eye/wp/2016/01/20/u-s-illegal-immigrant-population-falls-below-11-million-continuing-nearly-decade-long-decline-report-says/. Accessed October 10, 2016.

Passel, J. S. (2006, March). The size and characteristics of the unauthorized migrant population in the U.S. estimates based on the March 2005 Current Population Survey. Pew Research Center, Spanish Trends. https://www.pewresearch.org/hispanic/2006/03/07/size-and-characteristics-of-the-unauthorized-migrant-population-in-the-us/. Accessed October 10, 2018.

Pew Research Center, Social & Demographic Trends. (2013, February 7). Second-generation Americans: A portrait of the adult children of immigrants. https://www.pewsocialtrends.org/2013/02/07/second-generation-americans//. Accessed October 15, 2018.

Pumariega, A. J., & Rothe, E. M. (2010). Leaving no children or families outside: The challenges of immigration. *Journal of Orthopyschiatry, 80*(4), 505–515.

Rothe, E. M., Pumariega, A. J., & Sabagh, D. (2011). Identity and acculturation in immigrant and second generation adolescents. *Adolescent Psychiatry, 1*, 72–81.

US Census. (2014, June 23). Population reports. https://www.census.gov/prod/www/population.html. Accessed October 10, 2016.

Zong, J., Batalova, J., & Hallock, J. (2019, March). Frequently requested statistics on immigrants and immigration in the United States. Migration Policy Institute. https://www.migrationpolicy.org/article/frequently-requested-statistics-immigrants-and-immigration-united-states. Accessed December 25, 2018.

3

The Psychodynamic Aspects of Migration

The course of human life can be seen metaphorically as a succession of migrations in which the individual moves away from the early figures of childhood to form new attachments through the different stages of development (Grinberg & Grinberg, 1984, 1989). These migrations begin in the womb, and after the baby is born, the baby enters the world and begins the trajectory of life. The journey of separations continues when the baby is weaned from the mother's breast, followed later by the onset of locomotion, which allows the child to begin to move away from the mother and traverse the stage of *separation–individuation,* which is regarded as the *first individuation* (Mahler, Pine, & Bergman, 1975). A series of other migrations continue to occur, including the departure from the parental home after adolescence, which constitutes the *second individuation*; choosing a partner; forming a family; assuming new professional and social roles; and eventually facing old age and a gradual loss of productivity and sometimes a migration toward retirement. Finally, the person faces death, the last of the migrations.

Every migration involves loss, moving on, and forming of new attachments, so mourning is always involved. Migrating to a new land and leaving one's home country typically activates a mourning process. Immigrants mourn the separation from their loved ones, parents, siblings, and sometimes their own children. They also mourn the loss of their friends and their broader network of relationships. They mourn *a sense of place and belonging* and familiarity with the objects of everyday life, of a particular climate and geography, and departure or distancing from the early life experiences that have so much shaped their personalities. They may miss the familiar smells, foods, sounds, rhythms, and elements of the native culture that have been incorporated by the individual from their earliest preverbal experiences and interactions with caretakers (Ainslie, Tummala-Narra, Harlem, Barbanel, & Ruth, 2013). So, Akhtar (1999) has theorized that after the second individuation of adolescence, the process of migration can be understood as a *third individuation*. Sometimes, these experiences of separation, loss, and the encounter with the host culture are so powerful that Volkan (2007) has speculated that immigrants are, in fact, perennial mourners.

ARRIVING IN THE NEW LAND

In addition to severing important emotional attachments to human beings, places, and material possessions, the immigrant will have to adapt to the customs and language of the new host country, which will be compared to the customs and language previously acquired by the individual. Persons leaving their homeland and arriving in a new land are often faced with *culture shock,* which Ticho (1971) described as a sudden change from an average expectable environment to a strange and unpredictable one. In his now-classic paper, Mexican psychoanalyst Cesar Garza-Guerrero (1974) addressed the process of culture shock, which he described as an anxiety-provoking and violent encounter that challenges the psychic stability of the immigrant and, when it is resolved successfully, leads to emotional growth. He described two main aspects of culture shock: (1) mourning over the loss of emotional attachments and (2) the vicissitudes or gradual transformation of the immigrant's identity in his adaptation to the culture of the new land.

Garza-Guerrero (1974) described three different subphases of the mourning process associated with culture shock: (1) *the cultural encounter*, (2) reorganization, and (3) the new identity. The cultural encounter is characterized by suddenness, acuteness, and abruptness as the immigrant begins to explore the similarities and differences that exist between the culture of origin and the culture of the host country, as well as preconceived ideas and anticipations about the new culture. If the discrepancy is too great, puzzlement and disillusionment emerge, and anxiety, sadness, and confusion may follow, with a longing to recover what was lost. A jarring discontinuity occurs, and the immigrant struggles to recover, among other things, a sense of continuity of the self and an awareness of self-sameness, a sense of consistency of one's personal interactions with others and a sense of confirmation of one's identity in interaction with one's environment. All of these elements constitute one's own recognition of *who one is*, and they may come under assault during the process of culture shock, posing a threat to the person's identity. A vivid example of culture shock is illustrated in the following case:

Case I

Juan, an 11-year-old Puerto Rican boy, arrived in Boston with his mother and two brothers after his mother left the island abruptly when she discovered that her husband and father of the children was having an affair with the next-door neighbor. The family ended up living in the small inner-city apartment of the mother's sister with the sister, her 13-year-old son, and the children's maternal grandmother; soon, family tensions ensued. Juan was referred to the neighborhood psychiatric clinic by a pediatrician, who identified the boy as psychotic and experiencing hallucinations. On interviewing Juan, the psychiatrist learned that the boy was grieving over the loss of contact with his father and with everything that had constituted his familiar environment and described his hallucinations to the doctor: "I see a map of Puerto Rico appear in front of me, and I try to hold on to it, but it slowly fades away and gets replaced by one of the United States, then I become really sad and begin to cry."

Argentinian psychoanalysts Leon and Rebecca Grinberg (1984, 1989) wrote eloquently about the psychodynamic experiences of migration based on their own experiences of migration and exile from Argentina to Spain. They described three forms of disorientation that may affect the immigrant. (1) In *spatial disorientation*, the immigrant may become confused on waking up in the new country, thinking he or she is still in the old country, or the immigrant becomes confused and calls places of the new country by the names of the old one. (2) In *social disorientation*, immigrants are confused by persons in the new country and call them by names of individuals from the old country. (3) *Temporal disorientation* causes the immigrant to feel that persons, things, events, and places in the present become confused with those of the past. Once the immigrant realizes these misperceptions, a feeling of sadness and mourning takes place.

The second phase of culture shock—reorganization—begins once the initial shock of the cultural encounter is over. This phase is akin to the work of mourning, in which the immigrant experiences fluctuations between the desire to adhere to the old culture, with depressive, idealized remembrances and longing for what was lost as the mourning for the lost culture is slowly worked through. The work of mourning serves as an inhibitory force by which there is a gradual letting go of what was left behind and a slow and gradual acceptance of what is part of the new culture, and a new intrapsychic reorganization slowly begins to take place. Some elements of the old culture that are no longer useful are slowly let go, and elements of the new culture are scrutinized and slowly incorporated, leading to a re-editing of the immigrant's identity. A more realistic assessment of the new culture takes place, and a new personality emerges based on the immigrant's selective identifications with elements of the new culture, eventually leading to a harmonious reorganization of the personality.

The last phase of culture shock, the new identity, is not a final product but a continuous re-editing process leading to enrichment and growth of the individual's ever-evolving personality. A new and gradual feeling of *belonging* in the new culture begins to ensue, and even though elements of longing for the old culture may remain, they are no longer paralyzing or have an inhibitory effect in the process of acculturation. Alongside the various losses involved in migration, there is also a renewed opportunity for psychic growth because human growth implies a continual exposure to new experiences and the reorganization and reshaping of the self based on our human need to form new emotional attachments with others. In this process, new channels of self-expression become available, resulting in an enrichment of the self (Akhtar, 1995, 1999).

THE MEANING OF LANGUAGE

The experience of an immigrant who arrives in a new country and is unable to speak the language may be similar to that of an adult who is demoted to the level of a 3-year-old child, which is the time when children begin learning the syntax of language. One of the major problems immigrants sometimes face is difficulty finding their place in the new land, recovering their previous social position and the professional status they held in their native country. All the skills that the person had acquired until then are temporarily lost, and a deep narcissistic injury and feelings of vulnerability occur. Even later, when the immigrant has accomplished some mastery over the second language, he may still not be able to fully convey his actual talents and capacities as he is able to do in his native language. All of the experiences of infancy, memories, and feelings are stored in the *mother tongue.*

Greenson (1950) wrote about the connection between the mother tongue and the mother and maintained that in infancy, speech is not only a way of preserving the relationship with the mother, but also a means of withdrawing from her. He added that when a person learns a second language, the person learns the vocabulary and grammar in a rational manner, but that the accent, intonation, and rhythm (the music of the language) can only be incorporated by identification with the person's earliest figures of attachment and, most importantly, the mother's voice, which the baby recognizes only weeks after birth. Grinberg and Grinberg (1984, 1989) also suggested that sometimes a person speaking in a second language may feel like he or she is *in disguise*, and that sometimes, only in one's native language are descriptions of feelings, situations, places, and things experienced as truly genuine.

Case II

> A successful Cuban American executive who immigrated to the United States in his early 20s was living in South Florida, a completely bilingual and bicultural community. One day he told the psychiatrist: "I only like to speak English when I am at work, and I always prefer to speak Spanish in my free time. I associate English with formality and stiffness and Spanish with who I really am. Curiously, when I have to explain technical things, even if the other person is a Spanish-speaking or a bilingual person, the explanation automatically comes out of my mouth in English. On the other hand, I don't like to socialize in English because it feels to me as if I'm still at work."

In therapy, the function of language acquires particular importance in immigrants and people who speak more than one language, especially as it relates to emotions, expression, authenticity, and the use of defenses. For example, it may be easier to say certain things and express certain feelings in one's second language than in one's mother tongue because, emotionally, the patient is not as affectively connected to those feelings in the second language, in the same way that speaking in the native language may create a greater sense of closeness and intimacy with one's true emotions (Ainslie et al., 2013).

THE TRAUMA OF GEOGRAPHICAL DISLOCATION

Ahktar (2011) has written eloquently about the trauma that the immigrant undergoes after separating from the geographical world and the many elements of the nonhuman environment belonging to the country of origin. Akhtar highlighted several of these elements related to the separation:

1. *Separation from a familiar climate and geography*: A loss of one's familiar ecological environment causes a discontinuity and a sense of strangeness in the encounter with the unfamiliar. A deep sense of alienation can overcome the immigrant when faced with topography, climate, and vegetation that were not part of his or her formative environment. At first, some immigrants may react with euphoria and curiosity at the newness of the adopted surroundings, but often a sense of alienation and a feeling of lack of belonging eventually occur.

Case III

> On completing his professional training in an American northeastern city, the first author visited an esteemed professor and supervisor to thank him and to say goodbye before returning to his home in South Florida. He found himself explaining to the supervisor some of the reasons that compelled him to return home. On hearing them, the supervisor added jokingly, "You forgot to mention something you said to me during the first winter you were here, that this place was 'dark and cold.'" Then he added, "It's so interesting! Those were also the exact words I heard from another one of my students who was from Texas."

2. *The loss of valued personal possessions*: People who go away to school or immigrate are often unable to take all their possessions with them, and many of them are left behind. These possessions may constitute what are known as *linking objects* (Volkan, 1981), which serve as a symbol that connects the immigrant to the memory of a person, a time, or a place. In everyday life, it is very common to encounter a man wearing the wristwatch of his deceased father or a woman wearing the ring or locket that once belonged to her deceased mother. These linking objects provide a sense of closeness with a loved person who has been lost. Other times, an adult person may have kept a particular toy or item that connects that person to their childhood and to a time that is invested with deep feelings and memories. Losing mundane personal items such as one's wristwatch; a particular item of clothing; one's old teddy bear, doll, or stamp collection, which are invested with a sense of one's self and one's identity, can be distressing and can cause a feeling of discontinuity because it may feel as if one has been robbed of an important part of one's self. The loss of valued personal possessions acquires an even more dramatic significance in the case of exiles, who are forced to exit their home and their country abruptly, leaving behind the totality of their material possessions and losing in the process the symbolic links to their loved ones and to entire periods of their life histories.

Case IV

The first author was very happy to reconnect with an esteemed female colleague from his training days whom he had not seen or heard from in many years. Like the author, the colleague was also an immigrant. After her training on the East Coast concluded, she had moved away and had been living for a long time in northern California. On speaking with her on the phone, she immediately broke into tears narrating how she had recently lost her house in a forest fire. She explained that her father had died 2 years prior, and that all the memorabilia of her father, including material possessions, framed photographs, and all the photo albums from her childhood had been lost in that fire. She was inconsolable and explained that losing her house and all her possessions had been just as painful, or perhaps even more so, than the actual death of her father, who had been ill for a long time.

3. *Alterations in man–animal relationships*: Akhtar (2011) has focused on a very unique aspect of migration: the change that immigrants experience in their relationship with animals, especially when they migrate from an agrarian to an industrialized society. He explained that in agrarian societies the variety of animals can form a part of people's everyday existence, and they become daily companions, symbols, or metaphors for myriad human emotions and passions, as well as receptacles of erotic, aggressive, or fearful projections. The pastime of *cockfighting* is common in many parts of rural Latin America, the Philippines, and the countries of the Pacific Rim. In these countries, raising and training a rooster to become a *fighting cock* is considered a valued cultural tradition and an art, yet in the United States cockfighting is forbidden by law, considered a form of animal *cruelty*, and people who engage in this practice are often arrested and face legal consequences.

4. *Encounter with new utensils of living*: Over the years of growth and development, the person accomplishes mastery over the utensils of living, of tools and instruments that surround him; these also provide an orientational framework for the person's sense of place and sense of identity.

Case V

A 56-year-old male patient from the Dominican Republic emigrated from a rural area of that Caribbean island to New York City, where he lived and worked for more than 20 years. After the patient accomplished a degree of financial success and stability, he migrated from New York City to South Florida, looking for a place that was more geographically similar to his place of birth. In therapy, he told the psychiatrist: "I really dreaded those first years in New York. I remember that I had a repetitive dream that haunted me almost every night. In that dream, I saw myself travelling in subway trains that were always coming and going through dark tunnels. They were going in no particular direction, and they never arrived at their destination, leaving me in a state of anguish and disorientation. I would wake up sweating and in a panic, and those same dreams lasted for several years. Even today, when I am facing an uncertain situation or a major decision over which I am unsure, I end up having a recurrence of what I call 'my subway dream.'"

Like in this case example, in the process of migration, the individual may abruptly come into contact with new utensils and machines that are unfamiliar, facing an external reality that has not yet been integrated and that is discordant with the person's internal reality. These images of the new utensils of living, of things and machines, often acquire conscious and unconscious symbolic meaning for the immigrant and sometimes may take years to integrate.

DEFENSES AGAINST THE TRAUMA OF MIGRATION

If the immigrant is still mourning and is not ready to accept the realities of the new host culture, this may mobilize a series of defense mechanisms that help the immigrant slowly work through the trauma of dislocation (Akhtar, 2011). These include *repudiation, return, replication, reunion*, and *reparation*.

1. *Repudiation* occurs when the immigrant faces the pain of the losses and the difficulty of the mourning process that lies ahead and reacts by rejecting everything connected to the new culture and the new community. In this way, the immigrant feels he does not have to mourn because in his mind he has decided that, "I am not really accepting all this; it's just temporary and eventually I am going back." A different

and paradoxical presentation of this same defense mechanism may appear when the immigrant expresses the opposite, that is, an idealization and exuberant joy after arriving in the new country with denial of any vestige of sadness or regret about what was left behind. In these cases, sooner or later the process of mourning sets in, and the joyful idealization eventually gives way, sometimes in subtle ways, to criticisms about the new host culture and regrets about what was lost. These defenses are often seen in individuals who have been forcefully exiled from their countries of origin, and they stand in defiance, refusing to accept their loss. These individuals sometimes form communities where they nurture and maintain a type of "frozen culture," denying the passage of time and living surrounded by remembrances of an idealized world that no longer exists.

Case VI

> Julian, a 66-year-old Cuban patient arrived in the United States at the age of 13 as an unaccompanied refugee child. He had been sent away by his family at the height of the Cold War to avoid conscription by the government into a communist boarding school. He never returned to Cuba. Most of his closest relatives stayed behind and died of old age on the island, and he was never able to see them again. He told his psychiatrist, "I have now been in the United States for the greater part of my life, yet I feel like I have never really accepted that I am now an American. I feel as if I do, I am somehow betraying my Cuban identity. Many times when I am alone, I close my eyes and imagine that I am travelling through the city of Havana in a taxi. I try to picture all the streets and the buildings and every detail from the scenery that I remember from my childhood. I get very upset when I blank out on a particular detail and immediately go to books or the Internet to look it up and recover it. I want to retain and experience those memories time and again because I feel that if I lose those memories I have nothing."

2. The defensive fantasy of *return* appears once the defense of *repudiation* is given up. Replacing repudiation with a fantasy of return allows the immigrant to focus on accomplishing such goals as advancing in one's studies, educating one's children, or accomplishing financial stability in the new host country. The idea of return is often "postponed" with a series of rationalizations in the immigrant's mind, and it remains as a fantasy that is longed for nostalgically, frequently in times when the immigrant feels lonely, uprooted, or homesick. The fantasy or desire of the immigrant to "someday be buried in my homeland" is also a part of these dynamics. This topic is elaborated in more depth in Chapter 6, Transnational Identities, Pilgrimages, and Return Migrations.

The fantasy of return acquires a different significance for exiles, who are not allowed to return, such as is depicted in this heart-wrenching poem, "Exile," by the Cuban poet Julia Rodriguez Tomeu (1913–2005), who lived and died in Argentina.

There will not be a flower emanating its perfume over my grave
because there will be no grave.
There will not be a shadow of a winding branch over the marble
because there will be no marble.
There will not be a line written on the stone that will say
who I was and where I came from.
Neither will I be there, because by then I will no longer exist.
Not a flower, not a tree, not a line.
Nor someone to repeat what I once said
or remember what I once loved,
which is only "exile"

3. The defensive mechanism of *replication* involves re-creating the home country in the new host country by the inclusion of cultural and ethnic artifacts, music, and foods characteristic of the land that was left behind. In the same vein, the immigrant might chose to associate only with people who are native to his own country, to celebrate the ethnic festivals and holidays of the old country with compatriots, or to move to a part of

the United States that replicates the climate and geography of the native country. Some immigrants may sometimes choose to live in an ethnic enclave such as a Chinatown, Little Italy, or other ethnocultural community that exists in cities throughout the United States where the language of the country of origin is spoken and that maintain a type of cultural bubble that replicates *the old country*. It represents the immigrant's desire to lessen the pain of dislocation, but when the adherence to the old culture is too strong, it can impede growth.

4. The defensive fantasy of *reunion* refers to the immigrant's idealization or sometimes exaggerated desire to attach to anything that represents the old country, such as restaurants, cafés, cultural activities, and festivals. The fantasy of reunion underlies these activities.

5. The defensive mechanism of *reparation* sometimes represents an unconscious fantasy that, by emigrating, the immigrant *abandoned* the homeland and in turn hurt it. Many immigrants return to their countries of origin to make donations or to build a hospital, clinic, or foundation that will help those in need. In the process, the immigrant is sublimating a desire to *heal* the land and those who were hurt by having been left behind, as well as to heal himself. Also, the immigrant may be trying, consciously or unconsciously, to leave a mark in his homeland, to not be forgotten and to assert his existence, even though it took place far away.

In the course of their journey, not only immigrants but also essentially all human beings form attachments that are followed by separations, and all of these attachments are deeply remembered and remain important for the rest of the person's life. Many times, these separations are accompanied by fantasies of reunification, which also appear in the belief systems of many of the world's religions. Some of these concepts are exemplified in a fragment of the poem "The Brick," by the Uruguayan poet Mario Benedetti (1920–2009), who lived in several different countries as a political exile throughout his life.

. . . because when I return
and someday I will,
to my people, to my lands and to my sky,

I hope that that brick I brought at great risk,
to describe to the world how my house had been,
will last as long as my tough devotions
to my substitute-companion homelands.
That it will live as a piece of my life
and that it will be laid as a brick in another house

IMMIGRATION-RELATED SEPARATIONS AND THE CHILDREN WHO ARE LEFT BEHIND

Immigration sometimes destabilizes the family, leading to a series of family fragmentations and reunifications. Families from developing countries tend to migrate in a stepwise fashion, with parents usually arriving first, securing employment and sending back monetary remittances, leaving the children in the temporary care of relatives back home. These separations from parents constitute a difficult reality for many children and adolescent immigrants today. The Longitudinal Immigrant Student Adaptation Study (LISA) (Suarez-Orozco & Suarez-Orozco, 2001; Suarez-Orozco, Todorova, & Louie, 2002) included 385 early adolescents from China, Dominican Republic, Haiti, and Mexico who were chosen from 51 schools in Boston and San Francisco. The study revealed that half of these students had been separated from one of their parents in the process of migration. The majority of the separations (79%) were from the father, and these separations tended to be lengthy (more than 5 years) or permanent. These adolescents reported more depressive feelings than did the adolescents who migrated with intact families. The study also revealed that the feelings associated with separation were experienced as painful and complex; for many, the absent parent had become an abstraction. Reunification with the parents was riddled with contradictory emotions and feelings of disorientation, especially if the absent parent had previously been the primary caretaker. Some of these adolescents reported relief and joy at being reunited with their parents, while others perceived their parents as total strangers and mourned the loss of grandparents or other family members who had become the psychological parents during the parents' absence.

Mitrani, Santiesteban, and Muir (2004) studied Hispanic families in Miami who were engaged in therapy owing to having a substance-abusing adolescent hospitalized in a psychiatric inpatient unit. They found that 21 of these families had undergone parental separations during migration. Of these adolescents, 71% had separated from the mother or maternal figure, 24% from the father, and 14% from both parents. The average duration of the separation was 7 years. The adolescents reported a variety of experiences during the separation, which ranged from tender loving care by relatives, to abuse and exploitation. The majority of the time, the reunifications proved to be disappointing for both parties, and the adolescents found that the parents were frequently overwhelmed by their own problems and unable to acknowledge the losses or feelings of the adolescent. In the process, sometimes sibling bonds were strengthened, and rivalries ensued between previous caretakers and parents.

Child fostering is the name that has been given to the practice of leaving children in the care of relatives back home while the parent migrates to American inner cities with the goal of reaching the *American dream*, from which the children will later be able to partake. This migratory pattern is widely practiced by Caribbean and Central American families that arrive in the United States, yet this phenomenon has been poorly investigated, and very little has been written on the subject. There appears to be no stigma attached to this practice, and most parents tend to be poor and desperate and are mainly concerned about providing for the immediate material needs of their family. They work for years in American cities, sending financial remittances back home, and are often oblivious to the psychological impact that these separations have on their children (Imbert, 2002; Mitrani et al., 2004; Pottinger, 2005; Suarez-Orozco et al., 2002).

Case VII

Jovana, a 16-year-old adolescent girl from Honduras, was referred to therapy by the family court due to oppositional defiant behavior, truancy, running away from home, and sexual acting-out behavior with her boyfriend. She had been declared ungovernable by her mother. Jovana had separated from her mother at the age of 5 after the mother immigrated to the United States in order to find better job opportunities, which would allow her to send money back to the family. Jovana was raised by her paternal grandmother in Honduras and saw her father frequently, even though he had remarried and had a second family. Eight years after the separation, Jovana's mother felt she had enough financial security to send for her daughter in the belief that Jovana would have better schooling and better opportunities in the United States. Jovana was evaluated by a team of psychiatrists at the child and adolescent outpatient clinic of the city hospital. She presented as an angry, oppositional, and defiant adolescent who argued openly and passionately with her mother during the initial interview. Her mother had only negative things to say about her daughter and accused Jovana of being ungrateful for not appreciating her mother's enormous sacrifices, intended to provide her daughter with a better future. Once she was seen alone by one of the psychiatry residents, Jovana was able to articulate her despair of having been separated from her grandmother. She then broke into sobs as she told her doctor, "My grandmother is my real mother; I am afraid because she is old and frail, and she may die soon and I may never see her again. I hate the U.S.; I didn't ask to come here. My mother is never home, and I have no friends here. The only person that understands me is my boyfriend. If they don't let me go back to Honduras, then I want to go live with him. Can you please tell my mother to let me live with my boyfriend?" Jovana and her mother were seen in psychotherapy sessions separately and together, and after 3 months it was decided that at the end of the school year, Jovana

> would return to Honduras to live with her paternal grandmother and to be close to her father. Her mother expressed mixed feelings of guilt, failure, and having been betrayed by her daughter. Jovana, in turn, expressed relief at the possibility of being able to return to Honduras.

Many times, children in these circumstances who develop behavioral problems in the United States are returned back to their country of origin, which functions as a type of reform school, "so they will learn respect." Usually in developing countries there is more supervision from members of the extended family and more adherence to traditional and religious values, and there is less tolerance for conduct disorder behavior among youth.

Case VIII

> A school principal in the Dominican Republic shared with the first author that, "In our school we cannot afford to have more than two 'Dominican-Yorks' (the term used in the island to define Dominican children who have been born or raised in New York or other parts of the United States) per classroom, because more than two can turn your classroom upside-down."

Practicing as a psychiatrist in the Dominican Republic, Imbert (2002) described treating many of these children whose reunification with parents in the United States failed after the children developed severe behavioral and substance abuse problems and were returned back to the island. This author described the dynamics of these families by evoking the biblical narrative of the *golden calf*. In this narrative, Moses, who had led the Jewish people out of oppression, returns from the mountain with a mandate of God (the Ten Commandments) to find that in his relatively short absence, his people have already forgotten his teachings and have returned to idolatry. He explained that Moses represents the *spiritual and the intangible,* whereas the golden calf signifies the *tangible, the material, and the immediate.* In working with these families, both the parents who migrated and the relatives who took care of the children while the parents were away and who had become their *psychological parents* found it very difficult to see beyond the material needs and to understand the distraught child's emotional and psychological needs.

PSYCHODYNAMIC PSYCHOTHERAPY INTERVENTIONS WITH IMMIGRANTS

A more in-depth discussion of the treatment of immigrants and refugees is addressed in Chapter 9, which discusses treatment, but it is important to mention some psychodynamic considerations.

1. *Validating feelings of dislocation and facilitating mourning*: The therapist must be empathic about the loss of continuity in the patient's life and allow space for the work of mourning to take place. This may include holding back on making interpretations and allowing the patient to embark on narratives of longing and nostalgia and to utilize externalizing defenses where the new acquaintances and new surroundings are accused and blamed for the patient's pain and losses. The therapist must validate the feelings of loss and confusion, serve as a container, and provide a safe space where the patient can complete the work of mourning. The therapist must also be aware of the immigrant's transferences to the therapist, where the patient may hope and expect the therapist to behave like a figure of the patient's past or may cling emotionally to the therapist in a regressive manner. This indicates the immigrant's feeling of helplessness and loneliness and the hope that the therapist will protect and guide the patient through the difficult times in the manner a parent or dear friend would. These can also become negative transferences, where the patient expresses frustration and disappointment that the therapist has not been able to alleviate the patient's pain, confusion, and loneliness. It is also important to be aware of the patient's transference to inanimate objects in the therapists' office and their symbolism, which may open the

door to important psychodynamic material and help move the treatment forward.

Case IX

> A 66-year-old patient who immigrated to the United States as a teenager once told the therapist, "I love the sofa in your waiting room. I could easily fall asleep in it. It reminds me of the sofa that was in the newspaper office when I was thirteen years old. After I finished the newspaper delivery route in my bicycle, which started at five in the morning, I would go to that office at around seven-thirty to get paid and then go off to school. Sometimes I arrived early and had to wait until the person in charge arrived. Many times I fell asleep in that sofa, to be woken up by the manager, who liked me a lot and would smile, say something encouraging and give me a check. I was so proud of myself and I felt like the luckiest kid in the world, because I was, 'making it in life.'"

In addition, it is important to pay attention to the comments and narratives made by the immigrant patient about conversations with people in the *old country*, especially given the new technologies that allow instant voice and face-to-face communication with individuals abroad. These comments, which involve idealization, devaluation, or longing for the country of origin, may serve as a thermometer to measure the ebbs and flows that occur during the process of mourning and adaptation to the new culture.

2. *Following a developmental perspective*: Akhtar (1999) recommended that the psychodynamic aspects of the treatment follow a developmental perspective because in addition to doing the work of mourning and adaptation, the patient is also *moving ahead* in psycho-social development. The therapist needs to help the patient find new words to define his new experiences and his new surrounding reality, offering hope and encouragement and acknowledging the patient's progressive accomplishments and his increasing mastery over his new surroundings and his new life.

REFERENCES

Ainslie, R. C., Tummala-Narra, P., Harlem, A., Barbanel, L., & Ruth, R. (2013). Psychoanalytic views on the experience of immigration. *Psychoanalytic Psychology, 30*(4), 663–679.

Akhtar, S. (1995). A third individuation: Immigration. Identity and the psychoanalytic process. *Journal of the American Psychoanalytic Association, 43*, 1051–1084. doi:10.1177/000306519504300406

Akhtar, S. (1999). *Immigration and identity: Turmoil, treatment, and transformation.* Nothvale, NJ: Aronson.

Akhtar, S. (2011). *Immigration and acculturation: Mourning, adaptation, and the next generation.* New York: Aronson.

Garza-Guerrero, A. C. (1974). Culture shock: Its mourning and the vicissitudes of identity. *Journal of the American Psychoanalytic Association, 22*, 408–429.

Greenson, R. (1950). The mother tongue and the mother. *International Journal of Psychoanalysis, 31*, 18–23.

Grinberg, L., & Grinberg, R. (1984). A psychoanalytic study of migration: Its normal and pathological aspects. *Journal of the American Psychoanalytic Association,* 32, 13–38.

Grinberg, L., & Grinberg, R. (1989). *Psychoanalytic perspectives on migration and exile.* New Haven, CT: Yale University Press.

Imbert, S. (2002). El becerro de oro: Los niños dominicanos que se quedaron atrás. *Psychline, 4*(2), 36–37.

Mahler, M. S., Pine, F., & Bergman, A. (1975). *The psychological birth of the human infant.* New York: Basic Books.

Mitrani, V. B., Santisteban, D. A., & Muir, J. A. (2004). Addressing Immigration-Related Separations in Hispanic Families With a Behavior-Problem Adolescent. *American Journal of Orthopsychiatry, 74*(3), 219–229.

Pottinger, A. M. (2005). Children's experience of loss by parental migration in inner-city Jamaica. *American Journal of Orthopsychiatry, 75*, 485–496.

Suarez-Orozco, C., & Suarez-Orozco, M. M. (2001). *Children of immigration.* Cambridge, MA: Harvard University Press.

Suarez-Orozco, C., Todorova, I. L. G., & Louie, J. (2002). Making up for lost time: The experience of separation and reunification among immigrant families. *Family Process, 41*, 625–643.

Ticho, G. (1971). Cultural aspects of transference and countertransference. *Bulletin of the Menninger Clinic*, 35, 313–334.

Volkan, V. D. (1981). *Linking objects and linking phenomena.* New York: International Universities Press.

Volkan, V. D. (2007). Not letting go: From individual perennial mourners to societies with entitlement ideologies. In L. G. Fioroni, S. Lewkowicz, & T. Bokanowski (Eds.), *On Freud's "Mourning and melancholia"* (pp. 90–109). London: International Psychoanalytic Association.

4

Acculturation

Acculturation refers to the process that occurs when groups of individuals of different cultures come into continuous firsthand contact, which changes the original culture patterns of either or both groups. The encounter causes cultural diffusion of varying degrees and may have one of three possible outcomes: (1) *acceptance,* when there is assimilation of one group into the other; (2) *adaptation*, when there is a melding of the two cultures; and (3) *reaction*, which results in antagonistic contra-acculturative movements (Redfield, Linton, & Herskovits, 1936). Acculturation is a concept that applies to individuals living in communities other than where they were born, such as immigrants, refugees, and asylum seekers.

Today more than ever before, acculturation has become a relevant concept as a result of the phenomenon of *globalization,* which defines the sociocultural climate of the twenty-first century. Globalization occurs when there is an acceleration of movement of people, products, and ideas between nations. It is characterized by an increase in fluidity between the financial and political borders between countries, which in turn increases the complexity of the everyday problems that are faced by the inhabitants of the countries (Coatsworth, 2004). Another important aspect of globalization has been the increase in large migrations in the last decades, predominantly from poor countries to more developed ones, like the United States (Rothe, Tzuang, & Pumariega, 2010).

ACCULTURATION ACROSS HISTORY: CHANGING VIEWS

The history of the United States is a history of immigration. The massive migrations that have shaped the identity of the United States throughout its history as a nation have often given rise to nativist movements, whose goal has been to stop or decrease immigration. They are led by the previously settled inhabitants, who perceive a threat to their established customs or fear competition in their job markets. These fears are often enhanced by the high fertility rates found among immigrant minority groups and lower fertility rates found among the more established groups (Pedraza, 1996). These historical reactions contributed to the concept of the "melting pot," which asserted that the best way to enter into the American culture was to assimilate, totally renouncing the culture of origin and immediately becoming American. This model applied well to immigrants arriving from Europe in the 1800s and into the twentieth century. Most of these immigrants had similar ethnic characteristics and often Americanized their names.

The term *acculturation* was first used in 1936 by a group of anthropologists of the Social Sciences Research Council and became an issue of wide discussion after the burgeoning refugee and immigrant resettlement crisis generated after World War II. The acculturation process causes change not only in the immigrant but also in the receiving culture, leading to a process of *interculturation*. Immigrants often choose one of several acculturation strategies: (1) *cultural maintenance*, choosing the extent that cultural characteristics are important to maintain; (2) *cultural participation*, determining how to participate with members of the host culture or remain among themselves (Berry, 1997); (3) *integration*, equivalent to assimilation; and (4) *marginalization*, choosing to segregate from the host culture.

The United States is an ethnically complex society, so rather than understanding acculturation as a uniform and linear phenomenon, Portes and Rumbaut (1997) have proposed the concept of *segmented acculturation*. Their research has mapped segments of immigrants with different patterns of acculturation in the United States; these differences are determined by factors that are intrinsic to the immigrant as well as factors that are intrinsic to the particular area of the host country where the immigrant arrived. For example, an immigrant from a rural area in Cambodia arriving in Oregon has a different acculturation experience than that of an Eastern European professional arriving in a northeastern American city to further his professional training (Rothe et al., 2010, pp. 685–686).

The concept of acculturation has not been traditionally applied to groups whose ancestors were subjected to involuntary subjugation in their own land, such as Native Americans or other indigenous cultures, or to individuals whose ancestors were brought to the United States by force and subjugation, such as African Americans. However, many writers and theorists have begun to apply these concepts to these historical minority populations as they have moved from geographic and social segregation toward greater integration into mainstream society and in that process facing many of the acculturation processes and challenges faced by immigrant groups, including adapting to mainstream culture norms and losing traditional cultural values and beliefs. Acculturation is a more complex process for these populations as they often have to deal with historical trauma from past oppression, as well as recovery of elements of their traditional cultures lost in the process of enslavement and oppression at the hands of dominant cultures (LaFromboise, Coleman, & Gerton, 1993; Pope-Davis, Liu, Ledesma-Jones, & Nevitt, 2000; Walters, 1999). In some cases, acculturation and acculturation stress scales have been developed for African Americans that have tested validity and reliability (Joiner & Walker, 2002; Landrine & Klonoff, 1994; Snowden & Hines, 1999).

MODELS OF ACCULTURATION

Acculturation was originally conceptualized as a linear process that took place in a continuum in which the immigrant discarded the culture of origin and slowly embraced the values, practices, and beliefs of the receiving culture. Until the first half of the twentieth century, this is the view that predominated in the United States. However, since the 1980s cultural psychologists recognized that the fact that the immigrant may embrace the beliefs, values, and practices of the receiving country does not necessarily imply that the immigrant will discard those of the culture of origin. In response to this, Berry (1980) developed a model of acculturation in which the values of the culture of origin and those of the receiving culture are measured in two independent dimensions that coexist in the immigrant. These intersect to create four acculturation categories:

1. *Assimilation:* The person adopts the receiving culture and discards the values and customs of the culture of origin.
2. *Separation:* The immigrant rejects the receiving culture and retains the values and customs of the culture of origin.
3. *Integration:* The person adopts the receiving culture and retains the values of the culture of origin.
4. *Marginalization:* The person rejects the values of both the culture of origin and the receiving culture.

In this model, integration leads to the achievement of *biculturality*, which involves developing an identity rooted in the culture of origin but developing values that originate from both the culture of origin and the receiving culture. Such a blended identity is often expressed using hyphenated terminology, such as Mexican-American, with the first position granted to the culture or ethnicity of origin. Another term often used to refer to children of immigrants adopting a bicultural identity is that of *generation 1.5* (born in the country of origin and raised in the host country and its culture). *Enculturation* is a term used to refer to the process of selectively acquiring or retaining elements of the culture of origin while also acquiring or retaining elements of the receiving culture (Weinreich, 2009), a process that is certainly involved in *biculturalty*.

Biculturality is considered to be the healthiest form of adaptation, with the most favorable psycho-social outcomes, especially among young immigrants (Benet-Martinez & Haritatos, 2005; Coatsworth, Maldonado-Molina, Pantin, & Szapocznik, 2005). Studies have shown that bicultural individuals tend to be better adjusted and show better self-esteem, lower levels of depression, and more prosocial behaviors and are better able to compete in the receiving community (Schwartz, Unger, Zamboanga, & Szapocznik, 2010). However, other researchers have argued that biculturalism may not always be the most adaptive and desirable mode of adaptation for the immigrant. This concept may prove adaptive in communities that are bicultural, such as Miami, Florida, but may be more stressful and less desirable in monocultural communities, where there is a pressure to conform and to assimilate and where retaining elements of the culture of origin may be perceived as foreign and be frowned on (Sam, 2000; Van Oudenhoven & Eisses, 1998).

As discussed in Chapter 1, the degree of ease or difficulty involved in integrating the culture of origin with the receiving culture will be mediated by the degree of similarity or difference between the two cultures. These similarities and differences may be actual or perceived and will determine how much adaptation is needed to adapt to the receiving culture. For example, language plays an important role in this process. In cases where race and ethnicity are the same in the two cultures, speaking English proficiently will facilitate the process of acculturation into the United States. For example, even in cases when race and ethnicity differ, Afro-Caribbean immigrants from Jamaica report less discrimination and acculturative stress than Haitians who speak Haitian Creole as a first language (Rudmin, 2003).

MEASURING ACCULTURATION

Acculturation is a complex construct that presents a challenge to investigators because it encompasses socioeconomic, historical, political, and psychological variables. In the traditional linear model of acculturation, the components of acculturation that are assumed to change are language and cultural practices (Rothe et al., 2010, p. 692). As previously mentioned, the understanding of acculturation has evolved from a linear concept to a multidimensional process of interaction between the cultural–heritage community and the cultural–receiving community. In recognition of the multidimensional nature of acculturation, its study has become of interest to the fields of sociology, political science, economics, and the mental health sciences. The inherent complexity of how culture influences cognitive mechanisms and human behavior may help to explain the proliferation of acculturation measures and the lack of substantive reviews of the literature that evaluate the specificity and validity of these measures.

Escobar and Vega (2000) have concluded that little explanatory power is added to psychiatric epidemiologic studies by the inclusion of multidimensional acculturation scales. Instead, when conducting epidemiologic studies, the preferred language, the person's place of birth, and the number of years residing in the United States are frequently used as proxies for acculturation. They are used as dependent variables that have consistent main effects on problems such as drug use and psychiatric disorders. Preferred language and place of birth are also stronger predictors when using multivariate models to predict health outcomes. However, Schwartz, Zamboanga, Rodriguez, and Wang (2007) argued that the linear model of studying acculturation misses multiple dimensions that are involved in acculturation. For example, in terms of language use, these investigators proposed that some immigrants may identify with their culture of origin, yet not be proficient in their heritage language, such as many latter generation Asians and Latinos in the United States. Also, in terms of ethnic identification, traditionally most White non-Hispanics have identified themselves as American. However, with the changing racial composition of the United States, it is unclear whether in the future people who reside in the United States will continue to equate American with White.

Cultural values are assumed to change when the person undergoes a process of acculturation. Some of the values that have been attributed to certain immigrant groups are also common to other groups. Schwartz and colleagues (2010) argued that more than being characteristic of any ethnic group in particular, these values may be common to people who emigrate from collectivist, agricultural societies to individualistic, industrialized societies, and that it is important for acculturation measures to take into account the context of reception of the host country. For example, if the immigrant is arriving in a rural, possibly more closed, community versus an urban, possibly more open, community, the economic characteristics of the community and of the host country at the time of the immigrant's arrival will have an important influence in the context of reception, as will the job skills that the immigrant may possess or lack and whether these are valued in the host community at the time of the immigrant's arrival.

Biculturality does not function as a pendulum that moves from polar extremes of white and black, but one that has many shades of gray. It can vary from a model that involves synthesizing the elements of both cultures to the point at which the separation of the elements of each culture sometimes becomes indistinct or to a model of segmented biculturality, in which the immigrant keeps the cultural values, practices, and identifications of the heritage culture separate from the new influences. Schwartz and colleagues (2010) proposed that in future studies, to accurately understand and measure acculturation, six processes need to be taken into account: (1) the practices, (2) values, and (3) cultural identifications of the receiving culture and the (1) practices, (2) values, and (3) cultural identifications of the heritage culture (Rothe et al., 2010, pp. 692–693).

GENERATIONAL DIFFERENCES AND ACCULTURATION STRESS

The family is the bedrock in which the child grows and is nurtured, socialized, hurt, and healed and develops an identity. The immigrant child faces significant pressures from peers, receiving culture institutions (e.g., schools or churches), and popular media to assimilate. The alternative may result in social or economic marginalization. Acculturation stress is the adverse effect of psychological conflicts resulting from the process of acculturation, apart from the physical health and lifestyle effects of acculturation (Berry, 1997). This results from internal conflicts over cultural values such as those that result between the immigrant's pressure of achievement versus family relations and family loyalty and the pressure to assimilate to avoid discrimination, xenophobia, and margination; the loss of natural protective beliefs and values; the loss of extended family and kinship social support (especially moving from an individualistic orientation to an extended family–centered and collective orientation); and the strains over changing roles (gender, relational, etc.).

A common source of acculturation stress is intergenerational cultural conflict, more recently termed *acculturative family distancing* (AFD). These conflicts are set up by the immigrant youth's stronger exposure to receiving cultural influences and a greater cognitive flexibility that results in a rapid assimilation into the host culture, especially the younger generation's ready adoption of the new language, cultural norms, and particularly new expectations around gender and family roles and limits. In these contexts, immigrant parents have slower adaptation to the new cultural milieu, particularly as a result of the demands of economic survival or success; greater *enculturation* and social isolation; lesser cognitive flexibility leading to greater difficulty in mastering the new language; and fears of new parenting role expectations and of their children's loss of their identification with the traditional culture (and consequently with their family). The conflicts between home and external community environments around cultural norms and values become acted out, and these differences lead to intergenerational psychological and interpersonal conflicts, such as in the following case example:

Case I

Kathy (Ekaterina), an 18-year-old young woman, emigrated from Russia to Miami with her family at the age of 7 years. Kathy was referred for psychotherapy because of oppositional defiant behavior

> at home and difficulties getting along with her parents. Kathy shared with her Hispanic male therapist that she felt "very American" and added, "I feel embarrassed to take anyone to visit my home because my parents barely speak English, and they insist on speaking to me in Russian in front of my friends. It makes me stand out and feel different, and I don't like it. I just want to be a regular person, like everyone else. My parents don't make any effort to fit in; they just hang out with other Russian people, and they don't understand anything about my life; it's like they live in another planet."

This case presents an example of how language use increases the cultural dissonance between two generations of an immigrant family. This dissonance leads to a feeling of alienation in the adolescent, who lacks the necessary guidance and support that parents are able to provide during the adolescent passage.

Acculturative family distancing has been studied among both Latino and Asian immigrant youth and families and has been associated with an increased risk for youth substance abuse and conduct problems (Portes & Rumbaut, 1997; Szapocnik, Kurtines, & Fernandez, 1980) and more recently related to depression, anxiety, and even suicidality (Hwang, 2006). For example, in the traditional Latino family, mothers are the guardians of the family morals and traditions and acculturate slower than Latino fathers, who are usually out in the workplace and in connection with the receiving culture. A study revealed that Latino female adolescents experienced more discrepancy in gender roles between themselves and their parents than Latino male adolescents. These discrepancies led to increased levels of depression and poorer family functioning for Latino girls, but not for boys (Cespedes & Huey, 2008). Another study reported similar findings for Latino female adolescents, but found that bicultural stress and depression affected Asian female adolescents even more when both groups were compared with European Americans.

For some immigrant groups, Asian Americans in particular, there is the added stress of being looked on as the model minority, which has progressively been debunked but still casts long shadows (Romero, Carvajal,

Valle, & Orduña, 2007). In the 1960s, sociologist William Peterson coined the phrase *model minority* to describe Japanese Americans who had assimilated successfully to the United States, and in the 1980s, the media expanded this phrase to describe the triumphs of Asian Americans (Chang, 2003). Many Asian Americans take pride in this image, but however positive this portrayal may be, it can lead to stereotyping Asian Americans as a uniform group.

There is consensus in academia that this portrayal may be detrimental to Asian Americans in various ways. It can diminish the federal assistance that is allotted to this group, and it increases the pressure exerted by Asian American parents on their children (as well as internalized pressure and stress by the child) to perform at a high academic level in school, which can lead to social isolation and increased suicide rates (Leong, Leach, Yeh, & Chou, 2007). Among 15- to 24-year-old women, Asian Americans have the highest rate of suicide deaths (14.1%) compared with other racial groups in the United States. Asian American men of the same age have the second highest rate of suicide deaths, at 12.7%. Despite these alarming statistics and other mental health problems such as depression, there is still consistent underuse of mental health resources by Asian Americans across the United States (Lee et al., 2008).

Other minority populations suffer from the opposite problem: diminished expectations of achievement as a result of racial/ethnic stereotyping that can lead to ethnic self-doubt or self-hate, resulting in parental lack of support for achievement and underachievement by the child. This can lead to lower socioeconomic status and its resulting mental health problems (Escobar & Vega, 2000).

The opposite of AFD is *generational consonance*, which occurs when parents and children acculturate at the same rate or when the parents encourage selective acculturation among the second generation, such that the cultural harmony between parents and children is maintained, allowing the children to adapt to their new American reality. *Cultural dissonance* occurs when the second generation is neither guided nor accompanied by the changes in the first generation. *Consonant resistance* to acculturation occurs among isolated immigrant groups, such as exiles, that are strongly oriented toward return and view their presence in the host society as temporary (Pumariega & Rothe, 2010, p. 508).

ACCULTURATION: EPIDEMIOLOGICAL MENTAL HEALTH FINDINGS

Epidemiological studies on the mental health of immigrants have consistently demonstrated that first-generation adult immigrants have lower levels of identified psychopathology than the mainstream population and their children (Escobar & Vega, 2000; Oquendo et al., 2001). In analyses of data from the Epidemiological Catchment Area Study (Robins & Regier, 1991), less acculturated individuals were found to have a better mental health profile, individuals with moderate acculturation had medium levels of mental health, and more assimilated individuals had the worst mental health outcomes. Suicide was also less prevalent in the less acculturated group. Pumariega and Rothe (2010, p. 508) have summarized the hypotheses that have been proposed to explain these findings:

1. First-generation immigrants are naturally selected to be a more resilient group given their decision to emigrate against many odds, with the second generation being "softer" and less resilient.
2. First-generation immigrants suppress their mental health needs in order to subsume them below their more basic and immediate needs for personal and material/economic security. Once the second-generation immigrants are more comfortably established, they can then pay attention to pent-up mental health needs.
3. The second-generation immigrants may identify more readily with the devalued and denigrated concepts of their ethnic identity, adopted from the xenophobic attitudes of the host culture, which may lead to *ethnic self-hate* and higher risk for psychopathology (Escobar & Vega, 2000).

4. Family support may be strained for generation 1.5 and second-generation youth because of AFD. This relationship may be responsible in part for the higher risk of psychopathology among immigrant youth and children of immigrants.

A number of studies have demonstrated the impact of acculturation and acculturation stress on the mental health of immigrant and minority children and youth. Some of these (dealing with individual and family/community factors) are summarized next.

INDIVIDUAL FACTORS

A number of early studies have found associations between higher acculturation/assimilation and risk for psychopathology among the children of immigrants. These studies not only support the findings of a higher level of mental health problems in second-generation immigrants but also clarify the processes through which these generational disparities arise and can be summarized as follows (Pumariega & Rothe, 2010, p. 509).

- A greater degree of acculturation to U.S. cultural norms was associated with higher abnormal eating behaviors among Latina adolescents (Pumariega, 1986).
- Substance abuse is higher among Mexican-origin youth living on the U.S. side of the border than among Mexican youth living on the Mexican side of the border. Second-generation status, depression, being male, and cultural factors (lack of family cohesion, unsupervised time with friends, no religious ties, media exposure) and school problems were predictors of high risk (Pumariega, Swanson, Holzer, Linskey, & Quintero-Salinas, 1992; Swanson, Linskey, Quintero-Salinas, Pumariega, & Holzer, 1992).
- Suicidal ideation and attempts are more frequent in U.S. Mexican-origin youth living on the American side of the border

compared to Mexican youth living on the Mexican side of the border. Cultural factors such as lack of family cohesion, media exposure, nonsupervised time with friends, and no religious ties were associated with higher suicidal ideation, but not with actual suicide attempts (Pumariega et al., 2010; Swanson et al., 1992). The findings around suicidality in these studies, which were done among middle school and high school students on both sides of the U.S.-Mexico border, in many ways predicted the higher levels of suicidality found among Latino youth in another study, the Centers for Disease Control and Prevention (CDC) Risk Behavior Survey (Eaton et al., 2008).

- Latino children suffer from higher levels of anxiety than European-origin or African American children, with significantly higher anxiety symptoms in second-generation versus first-generation Latino youth (Glover, Pumariega, Holzer, & Rodriguez, 1999).
- Externalizing problem behaviors in Latino youth increase with increased acculturation, with that relationship mediated by the level of parental involvement, with more involvement by parents and more familiarity of the parents with the culture of the host country serving as a protective factor and the opposite serving as a risk factor (Dihn, Roosa, Tein, & Lopez, 2002).
- In a study of 285 Asian American youth, acculturation interacted with parent–child conflict to predict suicidality. The less acculturated Asian youth were found to be at greater risk for suicidality when high parent–child conflict existed (Lau, Jernewall, Zane, & Myers, 2002).
- In a study of Japanese, Chinese, and Korean immigrant youth, age, acculturation, and cultural adjustment difficulties significantly predicted mental health symptoms (Yeh, 2003).

Other studies have further reinforced the relationship between acculturation stress and psychopathology among immigrant youth. For example, Ethiopian immigrant youth were found to have rates of depression slightly higher than U.S. Whites (9.8% vs. 7.4%), but three times higher than their cohorts in Ethiopia (3.2%) (Fenta, Hyman, & Noh, 2004). Bicultural stress was found to be higher among Latino and Asian origin youth, and this was significantly associated with depressive symptoms, even after accounting for ethnicity, socioeconomic status, gender, and age (Romero et al., 2007).

In another study that compared traditional gender role beliefs between adolescents and parents, Latina teens reported greater differences in these beliefs than Latino male teens and higher levels of depression mediated by increases in family dysfunction (Cespedes & Huey, 2008). Also, among Latino youth, lower levels of ethnic identity have been correlated to risk for substance abuse, more acculturative stress, and lower self-esteem (Zamboanga, Schwartz, Jarvis, & Van Tyne, 2009). Lower levels of parental acculturation have been associated with antisocial behavior in Puerto Rican youth, in both Puerto Rico and the Bronx, although youth acculturation was not correlated to psychiatric symptoms (Duarte et al., 2008). Latino youth with higher English language fluency reported greater violence exposure and post-traumatic stress disorder (PTSD) symptoms than those with lower fluency (Kataoka et al., 2009). Acculturative stress in Latino youth has also been correlated with physiological symptoms, difficulty with concentration, and worry symptoms of anxiety, and those youth who reported more perceived discrimination accounted for a large proportion of the variance (Suarez-Morales & Lopez, 2009).

FAMILY AND COMMUNITY FACTORS

In the *second-generation* youth (born to immigrant parents in the United States) and in *generation 1.5* (born abroad but raised in the United States), the risk for mental health problems increases. The success or failure at adaptation for these youth is highly dependent on family and community factors and circumstances. For example, a study that observed the levels of integration of Latino immigrant adolescents demonstrated that those who maintained their parents' heritage and cultural practices while adopting the practices of the receiving culture fared better and were able to accomplish integration in both worlds. These adolescents reported higher levels of parental involvement, positive parenting, and more family support. In contrast, adolescents who assimilated to the host culture and abandoned the practices and culture of their parents reported the greatest levels of aggressive behavior (Sullivan et al., 2007). Extended parental separations due to emigration (discussed more at length in Chapter 3, The Psychodynamic Aspects of Migration) are linked to problem behaviors in Latino youth, and separations from mothers are particularly linked to depressive symptoms, especially for females (Mena, Mitrani, Muir, & Santiestaban, 2008). In Russian immigrant families acculturation stress was found to affect relationships between parents and children when the levels of acculturation between them varied (Birman & Taylor-Ritzler, 2007).

In immigrant families where parents were not as fluent as their children in the language of the host culture and where there was a need for *language brokering* (when the children act as interpreters of English for the parents in a variety of situations), there were higher levels of family stress, lower parenting effectiveness, poorer academic and emotional adjustment, and substance use in Latino immigrant youth (Martinez, McClure, & Eddy, 2009). In Vietnamese families, greater youth *culture brokering* (when the children act as interpreters of the differences between the parents' native culture and the host culture for the parents in a variety of situations) has been linked to less parental acculturation and more family conflict (Trickett & Jones, 2007). These findings support concerns about the adverse psychological burdens of placing youth in the positions of being linguistic interpreters and cultural brokers for their less acculturated immigrant parents (Pumariega & Rothe, 2010).

There is a substantial amount of research to support the role of AFD in the mental health of immigrant youth and families. Immigrant families who perceived higher levels of AFD experienced more parenting difficulties (Buki, Ma, Strom, & Strom, 2003), whereas those perceiving lower levels of AFD reported less family conflict (Farver, Narang, & Bhadha, 2002). In Asian immigrant youth who reported higher AFD, there was higher individual and family distress and risk for depression, with the quality of the parenting relationship between fathers and adolescents serving as a mediator (Hwang & Wood, 2009; S. Kim, Chen, Li, Huang, & Moon, 2009). Korean Canadian youth who identified with their traditional culture perceived their families as more supportive and less rejecting (U. Kim & Choi, 1994). Another study found that increased acculturation among immigrant mothers allowed the mothers to be more attuned to their children's life experience and related to higher maternal monitoring and lower conduct disturbance in their children (Liu, Lau, Chen, Dinh, & Kim, 2009).

HISTORICAL MINORITIES

For nonimmigrant historical minorities, there is similar literature supporting the impact of acculturation on the mental health of these populations. Gibbs (1997) had originally posited that cultural protective factors led to lower suicide rates among African Americans. More recently, Walker (2007) reviewed the literature on African American suicide and the acculturation literature to derive a possible explanation for increases in suicide deaths for African American men and apparent resilience for African American women. African Americans were believed to be unaffected by suicide because of protective factors (e.g., strong religious values and cohesive familial support systems) embedded in the culture. Acculturation was found to contribute to the weakening of these protective factors, with negative consequences for African American male suicide.

A study of African American college students found that perceptions of higher acculturation and lower social support were correlated with higher levels of depression and suicidality (Kimbrough, Molock, & Walton, 1996). Another study that included 130 college students of African descent found that as psychological distress increased, confidence about seeking professional services became more negative in the face of a desire to maintain traditional cultural beliefs (Obasi & Leong, 2009). In a survey that explored abnormal eating attitudes among in over 2,000 African American women who read *Essence Magazine*, the researchers found that the strength of Black identity was negatively correlated to a measure of abnormal eating attitudes, and many women described that as they entered the workforce they felt adversely evaluated in their appearance, which also negatively impacted their body image (Pumariega, Gustavson, Gustavson, Motes, & Ayers, 1994).

An extensive review of the literature on Latino and African American youth substance abuse revealed that the relatively lesser acculturation exposure by African American youth may explain why their substance abuse rates have been historically lower (De La Rosa, Vega, & Radisch, 2000).

A study of Native American youth found lower rates of suicidality among certain tribes that had higher degrees of social integration, with the highest rates of suicidality found among the tribes that experienced higher rates of change and acculturation (May, 1987). Another study of Native American youth found that the development of bicultural competence was an important aspect for preventive interventions for substance abuse (Schinke et al., 1988).

CONCLUSIONS

The processes of immigration and acculturation have an impact on all generations of the immigrant or minority family and often lead to a fluidity of household compositions that may generate distancing and conflicts among the different family members and potentially result in adverse mental health outcomes. Clinicians treating diverse populations, and particularly immigrants, their children, and their families, must be prepared to understand divergent, and often well-hidden, worldviews as well as difficulties with acculturation that may cause intrapsychic conflicts in the immigrant. These may also result in interpersonal and intrafamilial conflicts among family members that can interfere, among other things, with the completion of the child's developmental process and eventual emotional adaptation and socioeconomic success as an adult. Most important is to keep in mind that the adult immigrant of today will someday become the American of tomorrow, and that the children of today's immigrants are a generation that should be equipped not only to understand their parents' immigrant past, but also to successfully navigate their own American futures.

REFERENCES

Benet-Martınez, V., & Haritatos, J. (2005). Bicultural identity integration (BII): Components and psychosocial antecedents. *Journal of Personality, 73*, 1015–1050. doi:10.1111/j.1467-6494.2005.00337.x

Berry, J. W. (1980). Acculturation as varieties of adaptation. In A. M. Padilla (Ed.), *Acculturation: Theory, models, and some new findings* (pp. 9–25). Boulder, CO: Westview.

Berry, J. W. (1997). Immigration, acculturation and adaptation. *Applied Psychology, 46*(1), 5–68.

Birman, D., & Taylor-Ritzler, T. (2007). Acculturation and psychological distress among adolescent immigrants from the former Soviet Union: exploring the mediating effect of family relationships. *Cultural Diversity and Ethnic Minority Psychology, 13*(4), 337–346.

Buki, L., Ma, T., Strom, R., & Strom, S. (2003). Chinese immigrant mothers of adolescents: Self-perception of acculturation effects on parenting. *Cultural Diversity and Ethnic Minority Psychology, 9*, 127–140.

Cespedes, Y. M., & Huey, S. J., Jr. (2008). Depression in Latino adolescents: A cultural discrepancy perspective. *Cultural Diversity and Ethnic Minority Psychology, 14*(2), 168–172.

Chang, I. (2003). *The Chinese in America, a narrative history.* New York: Penguin Group.

Coatsworth, J. H. (2004). Globalization, growth and welfare in history. In M. M. Suarez-Orozco & D. Baolian Qin-Hilliard (Eds.), *Globalization, culture and education in the new millennium* (pp. 38–55). Berkeley: University of California Press.

Coatsworth, J. D., Maldonado-Molina, M., Pantin, H., & Szapocznik, J. (2005). A person-centered and ecological investigation of acculturation strategies in Hispanic immigrant youth. *Journal of Community Psychology, 33*(2), 157–174.

De La Rosa, M., Vega, R., & Radisch, M. A. (2000). The role of acculturation in the substance abuse behavior of African-American and Latino adolescents: Advances, issues, and recommendations. *Journal of Psychoactive Drugs, 32*(1), 33–42.

Dihn, K., Roosa, M., Tein, J., & Lopez, V. (2002). The relationship between acculturation and problem behavior proneness in a Hispanic youth sample: A longitudinal mediation model. *Journal of Abnormal Child Psychology, 30*, 295–309.

Duarte, C., Bird, H., Shrout, P., et al. (2008). Culture and psychiatric symptoms in Puerto Rican children: Longitudinal results from one ethnic group in two contexts. *Journal of Child Psychology and Psychiatry, 49*, 563–572.

Eaton, D., Kann, L., Kinchen, S., et al. (2008). Youth risk behavior surveillance—United States, 2007. *Mortality and Morbidity Weekly Reports, 57*(SS-04), 1–131.

Escobar, J. I., & Vega, W. A. (2000). Mental health and immigration's three AAA's: Where are we and where do we go from here? *Journal of Nervous and Mental Disease, 188*(1), 736–740.

Farver, J., Narang, S., & Bhadha, B. (2002). East meets west: Ethnic identity, acculturation, and conflict in Asian Indian families. *Journal of Family Psychology, 16*, 338–350.

Fenta, H., Hyman, I., & Noh, S. (2004). Determinants of depression among Ethiopian immigrants and refugees in Toronto. *Journal of Nervous and Mental Disease, 192*, 363–372.

Gibbs, J. T. (1997). African-American suicide: A cultural paradox. *Suicide & Life-Threatening Behavior, 27*, 68–79.

Glover, S., Pumariega, A., Holzer, C., & Rodriguez, M. (1999). Anxiety symptomatology in Mexican-American adolescents. *Journal of Child and Family Studies, 8*, 47–57.

Hwang, W. (2006). Acculturative family distancing: Theory, research, and clinical practice. *Psychotherapy: Theory, Research, Practice, and Training, 43*, 397–409.

Hwang, W., & Wood, J. (2009). Acculturative family distancing: Links with self-reported symptomatology among Asian Americans and Latinos. *Child Psychiatry and Human Development, 40*, 123–138.

Joiner, T. E., Jr., & Walker, R. L. (2002). Construct validity of a measure of acculturative stress in African Americans. *Psychological Assessment, 14*(4), 462.

Kataoka, S., Langley, A., Stein, B., et al. (2009). Violence exposure and PTSD: The role of English language fluency in Latino youth. *Journal of Child and Family Studies, 18*, 334–341.

Kim, S., Chen, Q., Li, J., Huang, X., & Moon, U. (2009). Parent–child acculturation, parenting, and adolescent depressive symptoms in Chinese immigrant families. *Journal of Family Psychology, 23*, 426–437.

Kim, U., & Choi, S. (1994). Individualism, collectivism, and child development: A Korean perspective. In P. M. Greenfield & R. R. Cocking (Eds.), *Cross-cultural roots of minority child development* (pp. 227–257). Hillsdale, NJ: Erlbaum.

Kimbrough, R. M., Molock, S. D., & Walton, K. (1996). Perception of social support, acculturation, depression, and suicidal ideation among African American college students at predominantly Black and predominantly White universities. *Journal of Negro Education, 65*(3), 295–307.

LaFromboise, T., Coleman, H. L., & Gerton, J. (1993). Psychological impact of biculturalism: Evidence and theory. *Psychological Bulletin, 114*(3), 395.

Landrine, H., & Klonoff, E. A. (1994). The African American Acculturation Scale: Development, reliability, and validity. *Journal of Black Psychology, 20*(2), 104–127.

Lau, A., Jernewall, N., Zane, N., & Myers, H. (2002). Correlates of suicidal behaviors among Asian American outpatient youths. *Cultural Diversity and Ethnic Minority Psychology, 8*, 199–213.

Lee, S., Juon, H. S., Martinez, G., et al. (2008). Model minority at risk: Expressed needs of mental health by Asian American young adults. *Journal of Community Health, 34*(2), 144–152.

Leong, F. T., Leach, M. M., Yeh, C., & Chou, E. (2007). Suicide among Asian Americans: What do we know? What do we need to know? *Death Studies, 31*(5), 417–434. https://aquila.usm.edu/fac_pubs/2104

Liu, L., Lau, A., Chen, A., Dinh, K., & Kim, S. (2009). The influence of maternal acculturation, neighborhood disadvantage, and parenting on Chinese-American adolescents' conduct problems: Testing the segmented assimilation hypothesis. *Journal of Youth and Adolescence, 38*, 691–702.

Martinez, C., McClure, H., & Eddy, J. (2009). Language brokering contexts and behavioral and emotional adjustment among Latino parents and adolescents. *Journal of Early Adolescence, 29*, 71–98.

May, P. A. (1987). Suicide and self-destruction among American Indian youths. *American Indian and Alaska Native Mental Health Research, 1*(1), 52–69.

Mena, M., Mitrani, V., Muir, J., & Santiestaban, D. (2008). Extended parent-child separations: Impact on Hispanic substance abusing adolescents. *Journal of Specialists in Pediatric Nursing, 13*, 50–52.

Obasi, E. M., & Leong, F. T. (2009). Psychological distress, acculturation, and mental health-seeking attitudes among people of African descent in the United States: A preliminary investigation. *Journal of Counseling Psychology, 56*(2), 227.

Oquendo, M., Ellis, S., Greenwald, S., Malone, K., Weissman, M., & Mann, J. (2001). Ethnic and sex differences in suicide rates relative to major depression in the United States. *American Journal of Psychiatry, 158*, 1652–1658.

Pedraza, S. (1996). Origins and destinies: Immigration, race and ethnicity in contemporary American history. In S. Pedraza & R. G. Rumbaut (Eds.), *Origins and destinies: Immigration, race and ethnicity in America* (pp. 1–20). Belmont, CA: Wadsworth Press.

Pope-Davis, D. B., Liu, W. M., Ledesma-Jones, S., & Nevitt, J. (2000). African American acculturation and Black racial identity: A preliminary investigation. *Journal of Multicultural Counseling and Development, 28*(2), 98.

Portes, A., & Rumbaut, R. G. (1997). *Immigrant America: A portrait.* 2nd ed. Berkeley: University of California Press.

Pumariega, A. J. (1986). Acculturation and eating attitudes in adolescent girls: A comparative and correlational study. *Journal of the American Academy of Child Psychiatry, 25*, 276–279.

Pumariega, A. J., Gustavson, C. R., Gustavson, J. C., Motes, P. S., & Ayers, S. (1994). Eating attitudes in African-American women: The *Essence* eating disorders survey. *Eating Disorders, 2*(1), 5–16.

Pumariega, A. J., & Rothe, E. M. (2010). Leaving no children or families outside: The challenges of immigration. *Journal of Orthopyschiatry, 80*(4), 505–515.

Pumariega, A. J., Rothe, E. M., Swanson, J., Holzer, C. E., Linskey, A. O., & Quintero-Salinas, R. (2010). Suicidality and acculturation in Hispanic adolescents. In L. Sher & A. Vilens (Eds.), *Immigration and mental health: Stress, psychiatric disorders, and suicidal behavior among immigrants and refugees* (Chapter 5, pp. 57–70). New York: Nova Science.

Pumariega, A., Swanson, J., Holzer, C., Linskey, A., & Quintero-Salinas, R. (1992). Cultural context and substance abuse in Hispanic adolescents. *Journal of Child and Family Studies, 1*, 75–92.

Redfield, R., Linton, R., & Herskovits, M. (1936). Memorandum on the study of acculturation. *American Anthropologist, 38*, 149–152.

Robins, L. N., & Regier, D. A. (1991). *Psychiatric disorders in America: The Epidemiological Catchment Area Study*. New York: Free Press.

Romero, A., Carvajal, S., Valle, F., & Orduña, M. (2007). Adolescent bicultural stress and its impact on mental well-being among Latinos, Asian Americans, and European Americans. *Journal of Community Psychology, 35*, 519–534.

Rothe, E. M., Tzuang, D., & Pumariega, A. J. (2010). Acculturation, development and adaptation. *Child and Adolescent Psychiatry Clinics of North America, 19*(4), 681–696.

Rudmin, F. W. (2003). Critical history of the acculturation psychology of assimilation, separation, integration, and marginalization. *Review of General Psychology, 7*, 3–37. doi:10.1037/1089-2680.7.3.250

Sam, D. L. (2000). Psychological adaptation of adolescents with immigrant backgrounds. *Journal of Social Psychology, 140*, 5–25.

Schinke, S. P., Orlandi, M. A., Botvin, G. J., Gilchrist, L. D., Trimble, J. E., & Locklear, V. S. (1988). Preventing substance abuse among American-Indian adolescents: A bicultural competence skills approach. *Journal of Counseling Psychology, 35*(1), 87.

Schwartz, S. J., Unger, J. B., Zamboanga, B. L., & Szapocznik, J. (2010). Rethinking the concept of acculturation: Implications for theory and research. *American Psychologist, 65*(4), 237–251. doi:10.1037/a0019330

Schwartz, S. J., Zamboanga, B. L., Rodriguez, L., & Wang, S. C. (2007). The structure of cultural identity in an ethnically diverse sample of emerging adults. *Basic and Applied Social Psychology, 29*, 159–173.

Snowden, L. R., & Hines, A. M. (1999). A scale to assess African American acculturation. *Journal of Black Psychology, 25*(1), 36–47.

Suarez-Morales, L., & Lopez, B. (2009). The impact of acculturative stress and daily hassles on pre-adolescent psychological adjustment: Examining anxiety symptoms. *Journal of Primary Prevention, 30*, 335–349.

Sullivan, S., Schwartz, S., Prado, G., Huang, S., Pantin, H., & Szapocznik, J. (2007). A bidimensional model of acculturation for examining differences in family functioning and behavior problems in Hispanic immigrant adolescents. *Journal of Early Adolescence, 27*, 405–430.

Swanson, J., Linskey, A., Quintero-Salinas, R., Pumariega, A., & Holzer, C. (1992). Depressive symptoms, drug use and suicidal ideation among youth in the Rio Grande Valley: A binational school survey. *Journal of the American Academy Child and Adolescent Psychiatry, 31*, 669–678.

Szapocnik, J., Kurtines, W., & Fernandez, T. (1980). Bicultural involvement and adjustment in Hispanic-American youth. *International Journal of Intercultural Relations, 4*, 353–365.

Trickett, E., & Jones, C. (2007). Adolescent culture brokering and family functioning: A study of families from Vietnam. *Cultural Diversity and Ethnic Minority Psychology, 13*, 143–150.

Van Oudenhoven, J., & Eisses, A. M. (1998). Integration and assimilation of Moroccan immigrants in the Netherlands and Israel. *International Journal of Intercultural Relations, 22*, 293–307.

Walker, R. L. (2007). Acculturation and acculturative stress as indicators for suicide risk among African Americans. *American Journal of Orthopsychiatry, 77*(3), 386.

Walters, K. L. (1999). Urban American Indian identity attitudes and acculturation styles. *Journal of Human Behavior in the Social Environment, 2*(1–2), 163–178.

Weinreich, P. (2009). "Enculturation," not "acculturation": Conceptualising and assessing identity processes in migrant communities. *International Journal of Intercultural Relations, 33*, 124–139. doi:10.1016/j.ijintrel.2008.12.006

Yeh, C. (2003). Age, acculturation, cultural adjustment, and symptoms of Chinese, Korean, and Japanese immigrant youths. *Cultural Diversity & Ethnic Minority Psychology, 9*, 34–48.

Zamboanga, B., Schwartz, S., Jarvis, L., & Van Tyne, K. (2009). Acculturation and substance use among Hispanic early adolescents: Investigating the mediating roles of acculturative stress and self-esteem. *Journal of Primary Prevention, 30*, 315–333.

5

Immigration and Race

INTRODUCTION: RACE AND ETHNICITY

The United States was once a country with a large White majority population and a small Black minority with impenetrable color lines, but over the past four decades, immigration has increased the racial and ethnic diversity in the United States. Along with increased immigration are increases in the rates of ethnic–racial intermarriage, which is transforming the American landscape into one with a growing multiracial population. Currently, 1 in 40 persons identifies himself or herself as multiracial, and this number could increase to 1 in 5 by the year 2050, which would move the nation beyond the traditional White/Black color line (Lee & Bean, 2004). These demographic changes have occurred due to the arrival of unprecedented numbers of Latino and Asian immigrants, and new demarcation lines for race are beginning to develop.

Fredrickson (1988) has defined race as a: consciousness of status and identity based on ancestry and color. Sociologists are beginning to wrestle with the question of whether today's immigrants are helping to blur racial boundaries or whether America's newcomers are simply crossing over the color line rather than helping to eradicate it (Alba, 1999; Lee & Bean, 2004; Waters, 1999). Previously, Italian, Irish, and eastern European Jews were regard as "*non-White*" but were gradually accepted as White to distinguish them from Blacks. After 1920, the cessation of the massive immigration from Europe that had begun a century earlier allowed for these groups to no longer be seen as a threat to the American population. They began to assimilate into the American economy, especially after the economic boom that occurred following the end of World War II (Foner, 2000).

In the second part of the twentieth century, Hispanics and Asians began to migrate to the United States in large numbers. When asked to define themselves racially, more than 40% of Hispanics chose the "some other race" category compared with only 1% of the non-Hispanic population, in part because many Latinos see themselves as deriving from more than one racial group. In contrast, first-generation biracial Asian children are most likely to be identified as Asian compared with subsequent generations. In their study of multiracial youth, Harris and Sim (2002) found that when asked to choose a single race, Asian White youth are equally likely to identify as Asian or White, demonstrating that the racial identification of Asian White multiracials is largely a matter of choice. A second finding revealed that when a second language is spoken in the house, the children were more likely to identify as biracial.

The census revealed that Whites account for 77% of the total U.S. population, so most individuals who report a multiracial identity also claim a White background, yet multiracial identification remains uncommon among Blacks. The Census Bureau estimated that at least 75% of the Black population in the United States has multiracial ancestry (mostly White), yet only 4.2% of American Blacks identify themselves as multiracial. The differences between Black racial self-identification with that of the Irish, Italian, Jewish, Latino, and Asian immigrants, or descendant of immigrants, lies in the historical legacy of slavery, discrimination, and oppression to which Blacks have been subjected and which continues to marginalize this group, suggesting that racial classifications have a strong cultural and historical component in addition to a biological component.

Gordon (1964) was the first who proposed the view that there is one unidirectional linear pathway to successfully assimilating into the nation's economic and social structure, and that acculturation not only preceded, but also was necessary for structural incorporation. In this assimilation process model, immigrants lose their ethnic distinctiveness, become ever more indistinguishable from the host society, and eventually adopt an American identity. This model was applicable mostly to the White–northern European immigrants who arrived in the United States prior to the 1920s.

In contrast, Portes and Zhou's (1993), in their important article on *segmented assimilation*, proposed three possible pathways to incorporation into the United States: (1) a straight-line assimilation into the White middle class (seen, e.g., among light-skinned Cubans in Miami); (2) assimilation into the minority underclass (seen among the Haitians in Miami); or (3) selective assimilation, by which immigrants remain immersed in the ethnic community and preserve the immigrant community's values and solidarity as a means to achieve upward mobility (e.g., among Punjabi Sikh Indians in Northern California) (Lee & Bean, 2004). Many of today's new Asian and Latino immigrants adopt a path of "selective acculturation" (Portes & Rumbaut, 2001).

BLACK CARIBBEAN AND BLACK AFRICAN IMMIGRANTS

Black immigrants in the United States today number 3.8 million, more than four times the number in 1980, according to a Pew Research Center analysis of U.S. Census Bureau data. Black immigrants now account for 8.7% of the nation's Black population, nearly triple their share in 1980 (Anderson, Lopez, & Rohal, 2015). During the period of slavery, there was limited migration of Black slaves from the Caribbean to the United

States. This began to change after the Spanish–American War of 1898, and among some of the initial immigrants were workers who had labored in the making of the Panama Canal. In particular, between 1920 and 1950 the number of Caribbean immigrants increased by 540%. The immigration reforms brought by the Immigration and Nationality Act of 1965 lifted the quotas of immigrants by national origin and replaced them with a system based on family reunification and employment, which further increased the number of Caribbean immigrants (Thomas, 2012).

Nevertheless, the recent growth in the size of the Black immigrant population has been fueled by African immigration. Between 2000 and 2013, the number of Black African immigrants living in the United States rose 137%, from 574,000 to 1.4 million. Africans now make up 36% of the total foreign-born Black population, up from 24% in 2000 and just 7% in 1980; virtually all are from sub-Saharan African countries, with only 1% of all Black immigrants from North Africa. The largest number come from Nigeria, with 226,000 immigrants, and Ethiopia, with 191,000.

Black Caribbeans often arrive with substantial social capital, which advantages them over other native Blacks in terms of material resources, such as income, education, and occupational prestige (Manuel, Taylor, & Jackson, 2012). Given their superior economic circumstances, Black Caribbeans are depicted as a "model minority" who are differently assimilated due to their elevated minority status (Thornton, Taylor, & Chatters, 2012, 2013).

Similarly, Black immigrants from Africa are more likely than Americans overall to have a college degree or higher. But, educational attainment varies widely by country of origin. For example, 59% of foreign-born Blacks from Nigeria have a bachelor's or advanced degree, a share that is roughly double that of the overall population. By comparison, just 10% of Black immigrants from Somalia have earned at least a bachelor's degree (Anderson et al., 2015).

Many Black immigrants are from Spanish-speaking countries. Among these, the Dominican Republic is the largest country of birth, accounting for 161,000 Black immigrants. Mexico is also a source of Black immigration, with roughly 70,000 Black immigrants. Some 41,000 are from Cuba, and 32,000 are Panamanian; 11% of the foreign-born Black population identifies as Hispanic. Currently, 49% of Caribbean immigrants identify themselves as Black, but among immigrants from countries such as Haiti and Jamaica, more than 80% identify as Black. Most Black Caribbean immigrants come from English-speaking countries, which gives them a competitive advantage compared to other immigrants when they arrive in the United States, and they are the least likely of all immigrant groups to be unauthorized immigrants.

In terms of refugee status, most asylees were from Cuba (91%) and Haiti (9%). When compared with U.S.-born Blacks, foreign-born Blacks are older, with a median age of 42 years versus 29 years for U.S.-born Blacks; they are less likely to live in poverty (20% vs. 28%) and, on average, have higher household incomes. They are also much more likely to be married (48% among those ages 18 and older vs. 28%) than U.S.-born Blacks, which is likely tied to their higher median age. Black immigrants are somewhat more likely to hold U.S. citizenship than all immigrants, 54% versus 47%.

Given that many Black immigrants are from English-speaking Caribbean nations, they are also more likely to be proficient in English compared with all immigrants (74% versus 50%). Black immigrants are also less likely to be in the United States illegally than all immigrants (16% versus 26%). Compared with the U.S. population overall, Black immigrants have a slightly higher median age (42 years vs. 37 years) and, among those 25 and older, are slightly less likely to have a college degree (26% vs. 30%).

In addition, Black immigrants are less likely than all Americans to own their homes (40% vs. 64%), and overall they have lower household incomes. In terms of education, immigrant Blacks ages 25 and older are also more likely than U.S.-born Blacks to have a bachelor's degree or more (26% vs. 19%). This share is slightly below that of the overall U.S. population, in which 30% of U.S. adults 25 and older have at least a bachelor's degree. However, the share with an advanced degree, such as a master's degree, Ph.D., or a professional degree, is similar among all Americans (11%) and Black immigrants (10%). Black immigrants hold degrees at a similar rate as the U.S. foreign-born population, 26% of the foreign-born Black population ages 25 and older has at least a bachelor's degree, comparable to 28% of all U.S. immigrants.

But, there are striking differences when comparing Black immigrants with Asian immigrants and with Hispanic immigrants. Among those 25 and older, 50% of all Asian immigrants have completed at least a 4-year degree; only 11% of Hispanic immigrants have done so (Anderson et al., 2015). In terms of levels of education, immigrants from Trinidad and Jamaica were the most educated and those from the Dominican Republic the least educated. However, once Dominicans arrive in the United States, their children make great strides in education, taking advantage of the excellent New York public school system, the city where Dominicans have established their ethnic enclave. Overall, Black immigrants (28%) are somewhat less likely than the overall U.S. population (31%) to have a college degree or more, but Black immigrants from Africa are more likely than Americans overall to have a college degree or higher. But, educational attainment varies widely by country of origin. For example, 59% of foreign-born Blacks from Nigeria have a bachelor's or advanced degree, a share that is roughly double that of the overall population. By comparison, just 10% of Black immigrants from Somalia have earned at least a bachelor's degree (Anderson et al., 2015).

Curiously, in spite of the educational advantage that Africans may have, Afro-Caribbeans are more likely to be active in the labor force than Africans, and their median earnings were 11% higher than American Blacks, in spite of having lower rates of high school graduates. Caribbean Blacks are more active in the labor force than native-born Americans and all of the other immigrant groups and are more likely to become American citizens than all other immigrants. Among some Afro-Caribbean groups, women were more likely to be active in the labor force than men. This was most true for immigrants from Jamaica, Grenada, and St. Kitts, where up to 73% of the women were active in the workforce.

The percentage of Caribbean children younger than 10 years old is less than half of the U.S.-born population. Many parents from the Caribbean immigrate alone, leaving children in the care of relatives back on the islands, and there is a significant amount of return migrations and shuttle migrations between the islands and the mainland, which causes parenting discontinuities and renders these children and adolescents vulnerable to mental health issues, such as conduct problems, substance abuse, and poor schooling outcomes. However, among Afro-Caribbean and African immigrants, extended family arrangements are more common than among U.S. natives (Thomas, 2012).

THE ROLE OF INTERMARRIAGE

In the beginning of the twentieth century, intermarriage between Whites and other groups was very rare, but today Whites intermarry at such high rates that only one in five Whites has a spouse with an identical racial–ethnic background (Alba, 1990; Waters, 1990). A recent National Academy of Science study noted that the multiracial population could rise to 21% by the year 2050 because of rising patterns in intermarriage, and as many as 35% of Asians and 45% of Hispanics might claim a multiracial background (Smith & Edmonston, 1997). The growth of the multiracial population provides a new reflection on the nation's changing racial boundaries.

Today, 13% of American marriages involve persons of different races, a considerable increase over the past three and a half decades (Lee & Bean, 2003). However, this seeming erosion of racial boundaries does not include all racial groups. For instance, about 30% of married native-born Asians and Latinos have a spouse of a different racial background, mostly White. In contrast, only one tenth of young Blacks married someone of a different racial background, and only 5.8% of Blacks married Whites (Perlmann, 2000). The intermarriage rates for Asians and Latinos are nearly three times as high as that of Blacks and more than five times the rate of Whites. Among married Asians and Latinos, 27.2% and 28.4% of marriages, respectively, involve a member of another racial group, typically Whites (Bean & Stevens, 2003; Lee & Bean, 2003). The comparatively higher rates of intermarriage among native-born Asians and Latinos indicate that as these groups are incorporating very quickly into the United States and not only are becoming receptive to intermarriage, but also are perceived by Whites as suitable marriage partners (Lee & Bean, 2004; Moran 2001).

Based on these findings, Perlmann (2000) described three distinct trends in interracial marriage in the United States: (1) Intermarriage for all racial groups has increased dramatically over the past 35 years and will probably continue to rise. (2) Intermarriage is not uncommon in the case of newer immigrant groups, such as Asians and Latinos (particularly among the young, native-born populations). (3) Compared with Asians, Latinos, and American Indians, intermarriage is still relatively uncommon among Blacks. The differential rates of intermarriage suggest that racial–ethnic boundaries are more prominent for some groups than for others, and that among Asians and Latinos, racial–ethnic boundaries are more fluid and flexible, and that prejudice is less salient for these groups. By contrast, the lower rates of intermarriage among Blacks suggest that racial boundaries continue to be more prominent between Whites and Blacks.

In spite of the fact that the U.S. Census Bureau estimates that at least three quarters of the Black population in the United States is ancestrally multiracial, mostly White, just over 4% of Blacks claim to be biracial (Davis, 1991; Spencer, 1997). What sets Latinos and Asians apart is that their experiences are not rooted in the same historical legacy of slavery, with its systematic and persistent patterns of legal and institutional discrimination and inequality that have existed in the United States since the first slaves were brought to America from Africa. Unlike African Americans who were forcefully brought to this country as slaves, today's Latino and Asian newcomers are voluntary migrants; consequently, their experiences are distinct from those of African Americans (Lee & Bean, 2004).

What is apparent from these statistics is that (1) the multiracial population seems likely to continue to grow in the foreseeable future because of increasing intermarriage. (2) Multiracial identification is not uncommon among the members of new immigrant groups, such as Asians and Latinos, particularly for those under the age of 18. (3) Multiracial identification remains relatively uncommon among Blacks compared with Asians and Latinos. (4) These patterns suggest that multiracial reporting is more likely in areas with greater levels of racial–ethnic diversity, largely brought about by the post-1965 waves of immigrants, particularly Latinos and Asians. (5) The increases in intermarriage and the growth of the multiracial population reflect a blending of races and the fading of color lines and perhaps a reduction in social distance and racial prejudice; these patterns appear to offer an optimistic portrait of weakening racial boundaries. (6) Yet, the continuing Black–non-Black divide could be a disastrous outcome for many African Americans. Once again, they would find that newer non-White immigrant groups are able to jump ahead of them in a hierarchy in which many Blacks, or at least those with less than a college degree, find themselves continuing to incur extreme disadvantage for structural reasons (Lee & Bean, 2004).

DISCRIMINATION, RACISM, AND PERCEIVED RACISM AMONG IMMIGRANTS

Large-scale studies indicated that 87% of African American adolescents (Seaton, Caldwell, Sellers, & Jackson., 2008) and 50% of Latinos aged 18–24 (Perez, Fortuna, & Alegrıa, 2008) have experienced discrimination in the past year, and that these experiences of discrimination can have psychologically detrimental effects on some of these youth. Fortunately, not all youth who experience discrimination are susceptible to its harmful effects. As previously mentioned, projected population trends in the United States indicate that the country is becoming less White, with the share of non-Hispanic, single-race, White population expected to decrease from 66% of the population in 2008 to 46% of the population by 2050 (U.S. Census Bureau, 2019). There is substantial evidence of discrimination on the basis of skin color for legal immigrants in the United States, with immigrants with the lightest skin color earning 16%–23% more than comparable immigrants with the darkest skin color.

Hersch (2011) argued that current population trends in combination with an increasingly multiracial population indicates that the hierarchy of racial groupings traditionally perceived in the United States may be replaced by a hierarchy on the basis of skin color, in which persons with lighter skin color have an advantage relative to those with darker skin color, regardless of nominal race. Hersch (2008, 2011) also suggested that racial stratification in the United States is moving away from the current biracial system to one more like Latin America, with three racial strata that are closely related to skin color, and that the darker a person's skin color, the lower he or she is likely to be on any scale perceived to be desirable in the United States.

Slavery and postslavery discriminatory laws and policies in the United States were justified by beliefs that Blacks were mentally and morally inferior to Whites. The residual of those beliefs remains more than a century after the abolition of slavery in the cultural portrayals that depict Black Americans with well-known negative stereotypes, including the standards of physical attractiveness that are based on European standards; thus, African Americans with lighter skin are viewed as more attractive (Adams, Kurz-Costes, & Hoffman, 2016). Younger African American children tend to respond to the socially imposed stereotypes that lighter skinned Black people are more desirable; however once African American children reach adolescence and acquire more sophisticated cognitive functioning and greater world knowledge, youth's increased awareness of race and racial discrimination might foster pride in Black skin or, alternatively, might lead to preferences for lighter skin because of awareness of White privilege. In terms of gender differences, in a study by Hill (2002), as physical attractiveness scores increased, there was a corresponding increase in lightness of skin tone for women, yet for men the link between skin tone and attractiveness was much weaker and not significant. Dark-skinned men rated themselves as more sexually attractive than fair-skinned men, suggesting that for men, dark skin may be perceived as an asset in terms of attractiveness. In contrast, light-skinned Black women were more likely to be described as attractive and intelligent. The gendered nature of *skin tone bias* is also evident in the beauty products marketed to women of color, with many geared toward making women look more phenotypically White skinned.

Hispanic newcomers, including many who are dark skinned, poor, and undocumented, have come to perceive the social distance separating them from Whites as more permeable than that separating themselves from Blacks and are engaging in distancing strategies that may reinforce this distinction (Marrow, 2009). American Whites living in rural areas have been the most isolated from historical and contemporary immigration, but African Americans are also present in larger numbers in some of these areas and the "American racial binary" remains strong.

Bonilla-Silva (2002) argued that in the case of Hispanic assimilation into the American mainstream, three possible outcomes can take place: (1) Some Hispanics are allowed to "become Whites" and are fully incorporated and assimilated (such as the majority of Cubans in South Florida). Others are assigned to an intermediate group as (2) "honorary Whites," and a third group is assigned to the group of (3) "collective Blacks." While some Hispanics may become Whites or honorary Whites due to their phenotype or higher socioeconomic status, most Mexicans, Puerto Ricans, Dominicans, and Central Americans are collective Blacks due to their racialized incorporation as colonial subjects, refugees from wars, or illegal migrant workers.

Still, some evidence points to a Black–non-Black divide. Regardless of skin color, Latinos (especially Mexicans) are closer to non-Hispanic Whites than Blacks in their attitudes toward Blacks, suggesting that many do not see themselves as collective Blacks (Lee & Bean, 2007). In contrast, Black–White biracials usually identify as biracial or Black, underscoring enduring constraints on people with African ancestry. Adding to this divide is the fact that the socioeconomic position of Blacks is usually weaker, and many belong to the poor and working classes, while only a few belong to the middle class.

In this way, Hispanic newcomers enter local contexts heavily influenced by the racial binary and its resulting inequalities. Sometimes when newcomers migrate to rural areas where population sizes are small enough that "everybody knows everybody," they discover that complete racial isolation is not possible (Jimenez 2008). So, in certain rural areas there is a "triracial color line" model in which dark-skinned, poor, and undocumented Hispanic newcomers all become collective Blacks, perceiving greater distance from Whites than from Blacks, irrespective of African ancestry. In spite of this circumscribed experience, most Hispanics, including many poor, dark-skinned, and undocumented Mexican and Central American labor migrants, are neither self-identifying as nor perceiving that they are treated equally to collective Blacks in everyday lived experience. Many Hispanics have come to perceive the social distance separating them from Whites as more permeable than that separating them from Blacks and are engaging in distancing strategies that may reinforce this distinction (Marrow, 2009).

RISK FACTORS AND PROTECTIVE FACTORS IN EXPERIENCES OF DISCRIMINATION AND RACISM

Emerging research suggests that both perceptions of discrimination and internalized racism (endorsement of negative stereotypes of one's racial group) are associated with poor mental health. This research is of great importance at a critical historic moment when "being Black in America" is being met with high levels of racism, which can have vast implications for a group for whom depression is most severe and debilitating and a group that already bears the brunt of persistent health disparities (Williams et al., 2007; Williams & Mohammed, 2009; Williams, Yu, Jackson, & Anderson, 1997). Racism can be conceptualized as existing in three levels: institutionalized, personally mediated, and internalized (Jones, 2000).

Institutionalized racism is embedded in the institutions that the individual encounters in everyday life. *Personally mediated racism* presents itself as intentional or unintentional discriminatory acts against people of color through negative interpersonal interactions and prejudice, including being followed around in stores, thought of as less smart than others, called names or insulted, and given poorer services. *Internalized racism* can be defined as the acceptance of negative attitudes, beliefs, ideologies, and stereotypes perpetuated by the White dominant society as being true about one's racial group. These three categories of racism are considered to be additive and synergistic.

The bio-psycho-social model of racism suggests that the psycho-social stress resulting from repeated and cumulative incidents of unfair treatment can trigger a host of negative emotional and cognitive responses, which can heighten risk of psychopathology, including onset of depression, conveying to individuals that they are different, devalued, and not respected in society. For example, studies have found that *everyday discrimination*, a form of modern racism that is subtle and ambiguous, is associated with increased risk of past-year major depressive disorder (MDD) (Williams et al., 1997). This finding is consistent with theoretical formulations of *interpersonally mediated racism* as a psycho-social stressor that increases risk of depression for people of color (Jones, 2000). Experiences of discrimination and racism have also been associated with other adverse outcomes, such as low self-esteem, poor life satisfaction, Hypertension, increased risk of cardiovascular disease, obesity, and shorter leukocyte telomere length (a biological marker of systemic aging), among others (Molina & James, 2016).

In essence, a substantial number of studies have demonstrated robust associations between *perceived discrimination* and poor mental health, with most outcomes focusing on psychological distress and depressive symptoms (Paradies et al., 2015). Previous research has shown that Afro-Caribbean persons in the United States have typically been regarded as "model minorities" compared to African Americans. Afro-Caribbean persons in the United States have, in general, higher levels of socioeconomic standing, including education and income and their numbers also partly comprise immigrant persons; all of these are known to be protective factors against poor mental health. Paradoxically, some studies have found that Afro-Caribbean adults report higher prevalence rates of lifetime depression and depressive symptoms when compared to African Americans. However, the effects of discrimination on mental health appear to impact these two groups in similar ways (Thornton et al., 2013; Waters, Kasinitz, & Asad, 2014). Molina and James (2016) analyzed nationally representative data of Afro-Caribbean (N = 1,418) and African American (N = 3,570) adults from the National Survey of American Life and found that among Afro-Caribbean respondents, but not African Americans, higher levels of internalized racism were associated with a *decreased risk* of past-year MDD. These findings were counterintuitive, but similar to previous research that showed that by acknowledging the stigma that is attached to one's ethnic group, the individual uses the stigma as a point of departure and defensively distances him- or herself from the assigned stigma in a self-protective strategy. In addition, *anticipatory vigilance*, a coping strategy that is characterized by monitoring and modifying one's behavior in an attempt to protect the self from anticipated racist events, can also serve as an effective defensive strategy to avoid the negative effects of racism. These investigators highlighted the complexity of analyzing these data and the risk of oversimplification, concluding that just as the Black population does not form a monolithic entity, the Afro-Caribbean group also does not, and that the decontextualized portrayals of Black persons in the United States (immigrants and nonimmigrants) may conceal important similarities as well as variations across cultural, demographic, geographic, and social dimensions. These differences are associated with divergent experiences, psycho-social adaptation, and different mental health profiles among Black ethnic groups (Molina & James, 2016).

Since the 1965 Immigration Reform Act, the United States has experienced an influx of unauthorized immigration, reaching a total of 12.2 million individuals in 2007 (Passel & Cohn, 2015). The majority (more than 65%) of these individuals have been Hispanic, primarily from Mexico and Central America. Unauthorized immigrants reside in the United States but are not citizens, do not hold a permanent resident visa, and do not have permission for work or residence (Cobb et al., 2018). Unauthorized Hispanics and other immigrants face not only challenges associated with being a minority in the United States, but also the additional burden of being an unauthorized immigrant; they have been portrayed in the media as unwelcome burdens in U.S. society. Together, these intersecting identities may exacerbate the perceived discriminatory experiences faced by this population.

Cobb et al. (2018) studied the risk factors and protective factors that mediated the negative effects of racism and discrimination in this group. They concluded that *ethnic discrimination* is a salient stressor for unauthorized Hispanic immigrants, but that a *high ethnic–racial group identity centrality* may protect these individuals from the negative effects of discrimination by providing a sense of belonging, acceptance, and social support in the face of rejection. When faced with discrimination, minority individuals can protect their well-being by increasingly identifying with their in-group, which may explain why ethnic identification tends to increase, rather than deteriorate, when individuals experience discrimination against their ethnic group.

So, it is not mere ethnic group membership that confers these benefits, but whether one's ethnic–racial group identity is *psychologically internalized* to form a central part of their self-definition and provide life with meaning. This is what is known as *ethnic–racial group identity centrality*. Such internalization of group membership is important because (1) it provides a cognitive framework for understanding oneself and one's place in the world. Also, (2) group membership provides a common perspective on social reality and furnishes individuals with increased feelings of belonging and purpose, providing them a better sense of control over their lives and more coping resources in the face of rejection, such as a sense of social support and acceptance. Finally, individuals with high ethnic–racial group identity centrality may be protected from the adverse effects of discrimination (3) because they perceive their in-group as not deserving such mistreatment, which has been also found among minority groups such as African Americans (Cross, 1995). In essence, empirical research has found that individuals with high group identity centrality report greater well-being, as indicated by (a) increased personal self-esteem and life satisfaction, (b) decreased depressive symptoms, and (c) improved cognitive health. In contrast, members with weak connections to the ethnic group will experience more adverse effects of discrimination because they lack a sense of social support, belongingness, and acceptance (Cobb et al., 2018).

It is important to note that there are significant differences between first- and second-generation immigrants in terms of how each group values the opinions of others. Perkins, Wiley, and Deaux (2014) studied the connection of *public regard* (the opinions expressed by others, in this case the members of the host culture, about the immigrants' ethnic group) and *private regard* (how members, in this case of the immigrant in-group, value their own ethnic group) and how both of these in turn affect the individual's self-esteem. These findings are important given that first- and second-generation immigrants make up nearly 24% of the population of the United States (U.S. Census Bureau, 2019). In essence, these investigators found that members of the first generation place more value on the opinions of members of their own *heritage group*, and members of the second generation (born in the United States to immigrant parents) pay attention to both their parents' heritage group and the host culture majority group, but place more attention to the opinions of the majority culture than to their parents' heritage group. In other words, when first-generation immigrants think of "others," they may be more likely to think of members of the heritage culture, having been born and raised in that context. In contrast, when second-generation immigrants think of others, they may be more likely to think of White Americans, having been born and raised in a context where Whites represent the dominant majority. In the case of immigrants of color, they are even less likely to identify with White Americans, placing more value on the opinions of their own heritage group. So, for second-generation immigrants and for immigrants of color in particular, if they perceive that the White majority group evaluates their group less than positively, they are at risk if they do not have a strong connection to their heritage group or their parents' heritage group. In turn, if they have a strong connection to their heritage group, they can decide to ignore the views of the majority culture group as a basis for their own regard and pay more attention to the opinions provided by their heritage group. If they think that people in the heritage culture evaluate their ethnic group in the United States positively, they also evaluate it positively themselves (Perkins et al., 2014).

RACIAL AND ETHNIC IDENTITY, ETHNIC–RACIAL SOCIALIZATION, AND CULTURAL ORIENTATION

Neblett, Rivas-Drake, and Umana-Taylor (2012) reviewed the literature that addresses the relationship between racial and ethnic identity, racial and ethnic socialization and cultural identity, and how they interact to provide resiliency to minority and immigrant adolescents.

Racial and ethnic identity: This refers to the youth's attitudes and behaviors that define the significance and meaning of race and ethnicity in their lives. Research has demonstrated that Mexican American adolescents who were faced with high levels of discrimination were able to maintain high levels of self-esteem if they had high levels of *ethnic affirmation*, while those adolescents with low levels of ethnic affirmation appeared to suffer (Romero & Roberts, 2003). In turn, African American youth with a positive connection to their ethnic group appeared to be protected against poor academic achievement and problem behaviors when faced with discrimination, while those who did not have this connection were not (Wong, Eccles, & Sameroff, 2003).

Positive identification with one's racial and ethnic identity appears to confer protection in several ways: (1) It may help to bolster self-esteem against some of the demeaning messages that are inherent in racial and ethnic discrimination experiences. (2) Racial and ethnic identity may make youth who experience discrimination less likely to make personal attributions (self-blame) for instances of discrimination, attributing discrimination to others instead, and thereby be less likely to suffer from damage to their self-concept. (3) The effects of racial and ethnic identity on youth adjustment may be mediated by coping skills. For example, individuals for whom race and ethnicity are more significant spend more time thinking about race, ethnicity, or discrimination and develop more varied and sophisticated coping skills that are more likely to lead to favorable outcomes and (4) that the youth's *sense of meaning in their lives* mediated the relation between ethnic identity and adjustment. So, combining meaning making, cognitive appraisal, and coping, in addition to a positive identification with one's racial and ethnic identity, promotes resiliency against experiences of racism and discrimination (Neblett et al., 2012).

Ethnic–racial socialization: Youth's racial and ethnic identity attitudes are often a byproduct of ethnic–racial socialization, a process through which caregivers convey implicit and explicit messages about the significance and meaning of race and ethnicity. They teach children about what it means to be a member of a racial or ethnic minority group and help youth learn to cope with discrimination (Hughes et al., 2006). Primary caregivers of ethnic minority youth differ in the extent to which they engage in ethnic–racial socialization, but several studies suggested that ethnic–racial socialization is fairly common across ethnic minority families. Some of the messages caregivers transmit to their children include the following:

1. *Cultural socialization*: teaching children about their racial–ethnic heritage and history and promoting cultural, racial, and ethnic pride
2. *Preparation for bias*: highlighting the existence of inequalities between groups and preparing youth to cope with discrimination
3. *Egalitarianism*: emphasizing individual character traits such as hard work over racial or ethnic group membership
4. *Self-worth messages*: promoting feelings of individual worth within the broader context of the child's race and ethnicity
5. *Negative messages*: emphasizing negative characteristics associated with being a racial–ethnic minority
6. *Silence about race and ethnicity*: failing to mention issues pertaining to race or ethnicity.
7. *Promotion of mistrust*: conveying distrust in interracial communications

Studies across diverse groups of ethnic minority youth link ethnic–racial socialization with a broad range of positive outcomes, including academic performance, ethnic and racial identity, socioemotional adjustment, racial ideology, ethnic affirmation, and positive self-concept. However, some ethnic–racial socialization messages can also have negative outcomes (Hughes, Witherspoon, Rivas-Drake, & West-Bey, 2009); for example, preparation for bias messages, in isolation, may contribute to low self-esteem in youth by instilling in them a sense of lack of control over their environment and leading them to disengage from academic and other pursuits. In contrast, patterns of racial socialization emphasizing both cultural socialization and preparation for bias buffered the impact that racial discrimination had on African American adolescents' perceived stress and problem behavior (Neblett et al., 2008), underscoring how various dimensions of ethnic–racial socialization coalesce to convey metamessages regarding the significance and meaning of race and ethnicity to youth (Neblett et al., 2012).

Cultural orientation: This refers to the youth's orientations toward mainstream culture or to their ethnic culture and has often been explained by endorsement of particular cultural values. Research on youth who have a strong orientation toward their ethnic culture described positive developmental outcomes such as good self-esteem, better academic engagement, positive racial self-image and psychological well-being, as well as less risk for substance abuse, depression, and externalizing behaviors.

Another similar concept that has been studied in relation to immigrant and minority youth and families has been that of *familism*, which encompasses youth's sense of family identification, solidarity, cohesion, and duty, as well as support received from the family. Various aspects of familism have been positively associated with psychological adjustment and its opposite, *acculturative family distancing*, which has been associated with deviant behaviors. Neblett et al. (2012) suggested that the three key factors of racial and ethnic identity, ethnic–racial socialization, and cultural orientation operate as protective factors against discrimination and promote youth adjustment; they reciprocally influence one another, simultaneously influencing and being shaped by self-concept, attributions, cognitive appraisals, and coping.

The *integrative approach* about how these concepts interact with one another is explained as follows:

1. All three constructs are found to contribute to ethnic minority youth's perceptions of their competence and adequacy and to bolster their self-concept.
2. Each of the protective factors may play a role in the cognitive appraisal process, including how youth attend to, understand, and make sense of the world. Ethnic–racial socialization processes prepare youth to perceive the world in a certain way, while ethnic and racial identity and cultural orientation may inform the salience and significance of discrimination in a given context, influence attributions of personal instances of discrimination, and provide youth with a sense of meaning.
3. *Coping* appears to be a critical intermediary process in the promotion of youth outcomes. Ethnic and racial identity and ethnic–racial socialization may facilitate the development of specific adaptive coping skills that help youth to negotiate ethnic and racial discrimination. Similarly, cultural orientation and values such as *familism* may provide the support necessary to help youth to cope. In addition, positive messages about the significance and meaning of being a member of a racial or ethnic minority group and positive feelings about one's group allow youth to feel competent across multiple domains and may inform how youth experience and understand the world.
4. Youth who are more aware of discrimination due to their identity, socialization, or cultural orientation may understand a racial or ethnic affront as part of the way the world operates, rather than as a personal derogation. Being able to make sense of their surroundings informs youth how to cope with their environment. Thus, youth who feel confident, capable, and competent develop more adaptive coping strategies than do those youth who feel insecure and perceive the world as threatening. In essence, it is likely that the protective factors operate in a cyclical, rather than a linear,

manner, such that they mutually influence one another across development (Neblett et al., 2012).

RACE IN THE PSYCHOTHERAPEUTIC ENCOUNTER

A small but emerging body of quantitative and qualitative research has provided support for broaching the issue of race and ethnicity during the psychotherapy process. It has been noted that therapists who demonstrate cultural responsiveness are consistently perceived by patients of color as being more credible and competent, and that therapists who actively acknowledged the importance of culture were perceived as being more credible by clients of color. In contrast, failure to address issues of race and ethnicity can perpetuate cultural bias by imposing a *dominant cultural imperative* on minority patients (Day-Vines et al., 2007; Gim, Atkinson, & Kim, 1991).

Knox, Burkard, Suzuki, and Ponterotto (2003) concluded that addressing race with patients of color occurred less frequently for European American than for African American therapists. In spite of this discrepancy, when race was addressed, both African American and European American therapists perceived these discussions had a positive effect on therapy. This collaborative exploration of racial dynamics enables the patient to feel that the therapist has an awareness of his or her sociopolitical experience, thus increasing the therapist's credibility with the patient. It is important that the therapist recognize the cultural meaning of phenomena described by the patient and to translate cultural knowledge into meaningful practice so that this ultimately results in the patient's empowerment.

The *therapy relationship* becomes the vehicle to navigate a discussion about issues of race and ethnicity that may be off limits elsewhere. In therapy sessions, this discussion fosters intimacy and forges a therapeutic alliance that can enhance therapeutic outcomes. However, in some cases, patients may harbor apprehensions about addressing these issues in therapy because of concerns that the therapeutic alliance may not represent a safe environment within which to disclose racial issues.

Many acculturated minority group members recognize that their survival depends on their socially conditioned ability to compartmentalize their lives, which many times includes negating the existence of ethnic–racial issues (Day-Vines et al., 2007). Often, this accommodation of *Whiteness*, whereby patients avoid issues of race unless prompted to do so, results from concerns about the power differential between the therapist and the patient in which the therapist wields the balance of power (Sue & Sue, 2003).

Racial identity functioning unfolds along a continuum from a minimal awareness of diversity to an increasingly integrated understanding and appreciation of the similarities and differences between oneself and others. So, sometimes the patient's reaction to the therapist bringing up the issue of race can serve as a diagnostic tool that provides implications for subsequent therapeutic efforts. Patients with low levels of racial identity functioning are likely to reject the therapist's invitation to broach the issue of race because they may possess low-salience attitudes about race. For instance, they may have other identities that assume more significance in their lives, such as their religious affiliation, sexual orientation, or occupational status (Day-Vines et al., 2007).

In broaching the topic of race with patients, Cardemil and Battle (2003) explained that with some patients the therapist should broach the topic by having a brief conversation and simply "putting the topic on the table" should it be relevant for the future. With others, therapists may find themselves involved in important conversations about the possible influence of race in the therapeutic process, yet with others the topic of race may develop slowly over time. The variables affecting how these conversations may develop include the level of the patient's trust in the therapist, the patient's understanding of his or her own racial–ethnic identity, and the overall importance that racial–ethnic issues have for a given individual. So, sensitivity to the appropriateness, timing, and pace of the conversations over the course of a therapeutic relationship is important. Taking all this into account, Cardemil and Battle (2003) designed the following recommendations:

1. Suspend preconceptions about patients' race–ethnicity and that of their family members.

It is important to remember that the racial–ethnic background of clients may not be obvious, especially when it involves biracial or multiracial patients or patients whose racial–ethnic identity is not obvious from physical characteristics. Similarly, patients who have a partner or other family member from another racial or ethnic group, such as in the case of adopted family members, may appreciate efforts on the part of the therapist not to make quick assumptions about the person in question's race because using inaccurate terminology may be offensive to the patient.

2. Recognize that patients may be quite different from other patients in their racial–ethnic group.

One significant benefit of engaging in conversations about race and ethnicity with patients is that it reduces the likelihood of stereotyping and the assumption that patients possess certain group characteristics. There is a literature that persuasively argues that all humans, including Caucasians, go through a process of developing a sense of racial or ethnic identity. For example, Sue and Sue (1990) proposed a racial–cultural identity development model where some racial–ethnic minority individuals move from an initial and self-deprecating (a) *conformity stage*, where the individual internalizes the identity that is imposed on him or her by the majority culture; going through (b) a *dissonance stage*, where the person questions and challenges the beliefs of the conformity stage; (c) a *resistance and immersion stage* that involves endorsement of minority views and rejection of dominant society; followed by (d) an *introspection stage*, less rigid in resisting dominant society views; and finally arriving at (e) an *integrative awareness stage* with an appreciation of the unique aspects of both the minority and the dominant culture.

3. Consider how ethnic–racial differences between therapist and patient may affect the psychotherapy process.

In addition to having conversations about the patient's ethnic–racial identity, it is important to acknowledge the ethnic–racial identity of the therapist. Many times, the patient will never raise this question explicitly; however, racial–ethnic differences may still play an important role in the therapy process. Such differences between patients and therapists may affect the psychotherapy process, including differences in attitudes and expectations toward mental health services and conceptions of the self in relation to family and community, communication and interaction styles, and differences in conceptualization of mental health and mental illness (Cardemil & Battle, 2003; Sue & Sue, 1990). Other cultural differences that may appear include (a) *different styles of nonverbal communication*, including *proxemics*, which is the way different cultures perceive appropriate personal and interpersonal space (e.g., hugging, kissing on the cheek, etc.); (b) *kinesics*, referring to the facial expressions, posture, movement, gesture, and eye contact among others; and (c) *paralanguage*, which involves vocal cues such as loudness of voice, use of silence, and pauses. All of these can lead to miscommunication and gradually infringe on the therapeutic relationship. For example, some Mexican Americans, Central Americans, and African Americans from rural areas and some Japanese may actively avoid direct eye contact as a sign of respect; a Caucasian therapist may interpret this behavior as a sign of shyness or guardedness, lack of assertiveness, that the patient may be hiding something and is not being honest, or that the patient has a depressed mood.

4. Acknowledging that power, privilege, and racism can affect the therapeutic process.

Many Caucasian therapists are certainly aware of these issues, but it is likely that minority patients will have experienced them more directly on a personal level. Moreover, minority patients may have had negative experiences in which the effects of racism, power, and privilege on their lives have been minimized or denied. Failing to acknowledge these societal issues in the context of psychotherapy could make the patient reexperience past painful personal experiences and thus alienate minority patients. In addition, *racist discrimination*, although illegal in the United States, is an unfortunate reality and continues to exist. Many members of racial–ethnic minority groups have had some personal experience of racism and prejudice in their own lives or in the lives of family and friends. For example, many African Americans report having experienced racial profiling by police conducting traffic stops, and many patients of Mexican or Central American origin may have been stopped by authorities to check if they are in the United States illegally. In addition to overt experiences with racism and discrimination, it is important for therapists to consider how *power and privilege* may influence work with racial–ethnic minority patients. *White privilege* refers to the set of advantages that are automatically afforded to those who share the dominant European American culture. Some examples of these *invisible privileges* include seeing people of one's own race–ethnicity well represented in film, TV, magazines, and other media and trusting that, in school, one's children will use curricular materials that contain images of people who look like them. Conversations about racism, power, and privilege can be difficult, particularly when a therapist is a member of the group benefiting from power discrepancies. So, it is more useful in these cases to explore how the effects of power, privilege, and racism may affect the therapeutic relationship.

Case I

A 55-year -old African American male gay patient narrated to his Hispanic American heterosexual therapist the humiliating experience he endured at the hands of a new primary care physician (PCP) in his plan who during the first interview lectured him about his herpesvirus condition, insinuating that this was related to sexual promiscuity. "The worst thing was that he did it in front of a medical student," the patient explained as he broke into sobs. After validating the patient's deep feelings of humiliation and the insensitivity and lack of medical professionalism on the part of the PCP, the therapist interjected, "I wonder if perhaps when you first came to see me you were worried that I would not be able to accept you and understand you as a Black and gay man?" The patient immediately acknowledged that this had been very much the case, and a discussion took place where the patient expressed many of his initial fears and apprehensions. From that point, he also became much more trusting and open with his therapist, which allowed the work of therapy to achieve new depths that may not have been possible if the issues of race and power had not been broached.

5. When in doubt about the importance of race and ethnicity, err on the side of discussion.

It can be difficult for both patients and therapists to determine when it will be useful to openly discuss issues regarding race and ethnicity in the course of psychotherapy. Some clients may address these issues directly; however, there may be subtle indicators that it is an important issue. When in doubt about the salience of these issues, Cardemil and Battle (2003) suggested that the therapist initiate a discussion in order to provide an opportunity for direct discussion should it be relevant because broaching the topic *directly and matter of factly* can convey a sense of openness to the patient, inviting future discussion on these issues as necessary. These conversations about race and ethnicity can be uncomfortable due to anxiety about offending or alienating the other person or being judged for "saying the wrong thing." In addition, some patients may simply prefer not to discuss race and ethnicity issues with their therapist. The more comfortable therapists are with conversations about race and ethnicity, the more easily they will be able to respond appropriately to clients who are themselves uncomfortable or uninterested in participating in these conversations. In the event that the patient appears uncomfortable when a therapist raises the topic of race and ethnicity, this can be approached in the same manner as when there has been an *empathic break* or a disruption in the therapeutic alliance. The therapist may say something like, "It was not my intention to offend you by bringing up the topic of race, but as we've discussed before, I want therapy to be a place where you can talk about anything that might be relevant to your life. In this case, I wondered whether anything related to our racial–ethnic differences might be affecting our therapy process."

Understandably, many therapists may still feel that raising issues of race and ethnicity with a patient in therapy is a risk they are not willing to take, no matter how much experience they may have. Nevertheless, broaching issues of race and ethnicity, even if the therapist is not sure of exactly what to say, is better than ignoring the topic (Cardemil & Battle, 2003).

6. Keep learning.

The United States has a long history of oppression of racial minority groups, and incidents of racism and discrimination still frequently occur. It is the responsibility of the therapist to learn more about issues of race and ethnicity, especially given the growing body of literature that has emerged about these topics in the mental health field in the last three decades. It is also important for the therapist to learn about the important sociopolitical events that have occurred in American history, as well as about issues such as acculturation and identity development.

We hope that this book serves as a reference source and as a useful learning tool.

REFERENCES

Adams, E. A., Kurz-Costes, B. E., & Hoffman, A. J. (2016). Skin tone bias among African Americans: Antecedents and consequences across the life span. *Developmental Review*, *40*, 93–116.

Alba, R. D. (1990). *Ethnic identity: The transformation of White America*. New Haven, CT: Yale University Press.

Alba, R. D. (1999). Immigration and the American realities of assimilation and multiculturalism. *Sociology Forum*, *14*(1), 3–25.

Anderson, M., Lopez, M. H., & Rohal, M. (2015). A rising share of the U.S. Black population is foreign born: 9% are immigrants and while most are from the Caribbean, Africans drive recent growth. Pew Research Center. https://www.pewresearch.org/fact-tank/2018/01/24/key-facts-about-black-immigrants-in-the-u-s/. Accessed September 12, 2019.

Bean, F. D, & Stevens, G. (2003). *America's newcomers and the dynamics of diversity.* New York: Russell Sage Foundation.

Bonilla-Silva, E. (2002). We are all Americans! The Latin Americanization of racial stratification in the USA. *Race and Society, 5*, 3–16.

Cardemil, E. V., & Battle, C. L. (2003). Guess who's coming to therapy? Getting comfortable with conversations about race and ethnicity in psychotherapy. *Professional Psychology: Research and Practice, 34*(3), 278–286.

Cobb, C. L, Meca, A., Branscome, N., et al. (2019). Perceived discrimination and well-being among unauthorized Hispanic immigrants: The moderating role of ethnic/racial group identity centrality. *Cultural Diversity and Ethnic Minority Psychology, 25*(2), 280–287. https://www.researchgate.net/publication/326426415. Accessed June 1, 2019.

Cross, W. E., Jr. (1995). The psychology of nigrescence: Revising the Cross model. In J. G. Ponterotto, J. M. Casas, L. A. Suzuki, & C. M. Alexander (Eds.), *Handbook of multicultural counseling* (pp. 93–122). Thousand Oaks, CA: Sage.

Davis, F. J. (1991). *Who is Black? One nation's definition.* University Park: Pennsylvania State University Press.

Day-Vines, N. L., Wood, S. M., Grothaus, T., et al. (2007). Broaching the subjects of race, ethnicity, and culture during the counseling process. *Journal of Counseling & Development. 85*, 401–409.

Foner, N. (2000). *From Ellis Island to JFK: New York's Two great waves of immigration.* New Haven, CT/New York: Yale University Press/Russell Sage Foundation.

Fredrickson, G. M. (1988). *The arrogance of race: Historical perspectives on slavery, racism, and social inequality.* Middletown, CT: Wesleyan University Press.

Gim, R., Atkinson, D., & Kim, S. (1991). Asian-American acculturation, counselor ethnicity and cultural sensitivity, and ratings of counselors. *Journal of Counseling Psychology, 38*, 57–62.

Gordon, M. (1964). *Assimilation in American life.* New York: Oxford University Press.

Harris, D. R., & Sim, J. J. (2002). Who is multiracial? Assessing the complexity of lived race. *American Sociological Review, 67*(4), 614–627.

Hersch, J. (2008). Profiling the new immigrant worker: The effects of skin color and height. *Journal of Labor Economics, 26*(2), 345–386.

Hersch, J. (2011). The persistence of skin color discrimination for immigrants. *Social Science Research, 40*, 1337–1349.

Hill, M. (2002). Skin color and the perception of attractiveness among African Americans: Does gender make a difference? *Social Psychology Quarterly, 65*, 77–91.

Hughes, D., Rodriguez, J., Smith, E. P., Johnson, D. J., Stevenson, H. C., & Spicer, P. (2006). Parents' ethnic-racial socialization practices: A review of research and directions for future study. *Developmental Psychology, 42*, 747–770.

Hughes, D., Witherspoon, D., Rivas-Drake, D., & West-Bey, N. (2009). Received ethnic-racial socialization messages and youth's academic and behavioral outcomes: Examining the mediating role of ethnic identity and self-esteem. *Cultural Diversity and Ethnic Minority Psychology, 15*, 112–124.

Jimenez, T. R. (2008). Mexican-immigrant replenishment and the continuing significance of ethnicity and race. *American Journal of Sociology, 113*(6), 1527–1567.

Jones, C. P. (2000). Levels of racism: A theoretic framework and a gardener's tale. *American Journal of Public Health, 90*, 1212–1215.

Knox, S., Burkard, A. W., Suzuki, L. A., & Ponterotto, J. G. (2003). African American and European American therapists' experiences of addressing race and cross-racial psychotherapy dyads. *Journal of Counseling Psychology, 50*, 466–481.

Lee, J., & Bean, F. D. (2003). Beyond Black and White: Remaking race in America. *Contexts, 2*(3), 26–33.

Lee, J., & Bean, F. D. (2004). America's changing color lines: Immigration, race/ethnicity, and multiracial identification. *Annual Review of Sociology, 30*, 221–242.

Lee, J., & Bean, F. D. (2007). Reinventing the color line: Immigration and America's new racial/ethnic divide. *Social Forces, 86*(2), 561–586.

Manuel, R., Taylor, R. J., & Jackson, J. S. (2012). Race and ethnic group differences in socio-economic status: Black Caribbeans, African Americans and non-Hispanic Whites in the United States. *Western Journal of Black Studies, 36*, 228–239.

Marrow, H. B. (2009). New immigrant destinations and the American colour line. *Ethnic and Racial Studies, 32*(6), 1037–1057.

Molina, K. M., & James, D. (2016). Discrimination, internalized racism, and depression: A comparative study of African American and Afro-Caribbean adults in the U.S. *Group Processes & Intergroup Relations, 19*(4), 439–461.

Moran, R. F. (2001). *Interracial intimacy: The regulation of race and romance*. Chicago: University of Chicago Press.

Neblett, E. W., Rivas-Drake, D., & Umana-Taylor, A. J. (2012). The promise of racial and ethnic protective factors in promoting ethnic minority youth development. *Child Development Perspectives, 6*(3), 295–303.

Neblett, E. W., White, R. L., Ford, K. R., Philip, C. L., Nguyen, H. X., & Sellers, R. M. (2008). Patterns of racial socialization and psychological adjustment: Can parental communications about race reduce the impact of racial discrimination? *Journal of Research on Adolescence, 18*, 477–515.

Paradies, Y., Ben, J., Denson, N., et al. (2015). *Racism as a determinant of health: A systematic review and meta- analysis. PLoS One, 10*, e0138511. doi:10.1371/journal.pone.0138511. https://journals.plos.org/plosone/article?id=10.1371/journal.pone.0138511

Passel, J. S., & Cohn, D. (2015). *Unauthorized immigrant population stable for half a decade*. Washington, D.C.: Pew Hispanic Center.

Perez, D., Fortuna, L., & Alegrıa, M. (2008). Prevalence and correlates of everyday discrimination among U.S. Latinos. *Journal of Community Psychology, 36*, 421–433.

Perkins, K., Wiley, S., & Deaux, K. (2014). Through which looking glass? Distinct sources of public regard and self-esteem among first- and second-generation immigrants of color. *Cultural Diversity and Ethnic Minority Psychology, 20*(2), 213–219.

Perlmann, J. (2000). Reflecting the changing face of America: Multiracials, racial classification, and American intermarriage. In W. Sollars (Ed.), *Interracialism: Black-White intermarriage in American history, literature, and law* (pp. 506–533). New York: Oxford University Press.

Portes, A., & Rumbaut, R. G. (2001). *Legacies: The story of the immigrant second generation*. Berkeley: University of California Press.

Portes, A., & Zhou, M. (1993) The new second generation: Segmented assimilation and its variants. *The Annals of the American Academy of Political & Social Science, 530*, 74–96.

Romero, A. J., & Roberts, R. E. (2003). The impact of multiple dimensions of ethnic identity on discrimination and adolescents' self-esteem. *Journal of Applied Social Psychology, 33*, 2288–2305.

Seaton, E. K., Caldwell, C. H., Sellers, R. M., & Jackson, J. S. (2008). The prevalence of perceived discrimination among African American and Caribbean Black youth. *Developmental Psychology, 44*, 1288–1297.

Smith, J. P., & Edmonston, B. (1997). *The new Americans*. Washington, D.C.: National Academies Press.

Spencer, J. M. (1997). *The new colored people: The mixed-race movement in America*. New York: New York University Press.

Sue, D. W., & Sue, D. (1990). *Counseling the culturally different: Theory and practice*. 2nd ed. New York: Wiley.

Sue, D. W., & Sue, D. (2003). *Counseling the culturally diverse: Theory and practice*. 4th ed. New York: Wiley.

Thomas, K. J. A. (2012). A demographic profile of Black Caribbean immigrants in the United States. Migration Policy Institute. https://www.migrationpolicy.org/research/CBI-demographic-profile-black-caribbean-immigrants. Accessed September 12, 2019.

Thornton, M. C., Taylor, R., & Chatters, L. M. (2012). African American, Black Caribbean and non-Hispanic White feelings of closeness toward other racial and ethnic groups. *Journal of Black Studies, 43*(7), 749–772.

Thornton, M. C., Taylor, R. J., & Chatters, L. M. (2013). African American and Black Caribbean mutual feelings of closeness: Findings from a National Probability Survey. *Journal of Black Studies, 44*, 798–828.

U.S. Census Bureau. (2019). Quick Facts. United States. https://www.census.gov/https://www.census.gov/quickfacts/fact/table/US/INC110217

Waters, M. C. (1990). *Ethnic options: Choosing identities in America*. Berkeley: University of California Press.

Waters, M. C. (1999). *Black identities: West Indian immigrant dreams and American realities*. Cambridge, MA: Harvard University Press.

Waters, M. C., Kasinitz, P., & Asad, L. A. (2014). Immigrants and African Americans. *Annual Review of Sociology, 40*, 369–390.

Williams, D. R., Gonzalez, H. M., Neighbors, H., et al. (2007). Prevalence and distribution of major depressive disorder in African Americans, Caribbean Blacks, and non-Hispanic Whites: Results from the National Survey of American Life. *Archives of General Psychiatry, 64*, 305–315.

Williams, D. R., & Mohammed, S. A. (2009). Discrimination and racial disparities in health: Evidence and needed research. *Journal of Behavioral Medicine, 32*, 20–47.

Williams, D. R., Yu, Y., Jackson, J. S., & Anderson, N. B. (1997). Racial differences in physical and mental health socio-economic status, stress and discrimination. *Journal of Health Psychology, 2*, 335–351.

Wong, C. A., Eccles, J. S., & Sameroff, A. (2003). The influence of ethnic discrimination and ethnic identification on African American adolescents' school and socioemotional adjustment. *Journal of Personality, 71*, 1197–1232.

6

Refugees and Special Populations

Refugees are people who have been forced to leave their homelands due to persecution, war, or natural disasters; they face a threat to their individual safety or the safety of their family or community and seek asylum in other countries. In popular parlance, those who are victims of calamities ranging from famine to earthquakes and sudden storms, hurricanes, tornadoes, tsunamis, and floods are also called refugees, but the term is more commonly used to refer to those who fit the formal definition recognized by the United Nations High Commission for Refugees (UNHCR, 2016), that is, as border crossers *with a well-founded fear of persecution*, in other words, those who are *forcibly displaced*. In addition to those who do find a way to cross into other lands, there are many who cannot exit from their beleaguered countries and are known as *internally displaced persons* (IDPs). Their plight is in many ways the most precarious of all for they often remain captives of the very regimes that may have driven them from their homes and otherwise sought ways to oppress them through humiliation, ostracism, mass internment, and, in some cases, mass murder (Rose, 2014). Refugee status protects a person from being returned to his or her country of origin. The term *asylum seeker* describes an individual who has crossed an international border in search of safety and is trying to obtain refugee status in another country. For the purposes of this chapter, the term *refugee* is also be used to include asylum seekers (Ehntholt & Yule, 2006; UNHCR, 2016).

Experiences of war, persecution, violence, torture, participation in killing, disruption of attachments, and emotional losses increase the risk for psychological distress and may contribute to the risk of developing psychiatric disorders, especially in child and adolescent refugees (Hodes, 1998; Rousseau, 1995). The mental health literature on adult and child refugees has been concentrated on the diagnosis and treatment of post-traumatic stress disorder (PTSD) and now constitutes a separate field of investigation (Hodes & Tolmac, 2005; Kinzie, 2006). In spite of this, there is still a lack of accurate data on the mental health status of adult or younger refugees, and there is very limited information in their help seeking and service utilization (De Antiss, Ziaian, Procter, Warland, & Baghurst, 2009; Phan, 2000; Pumariega, Rothe, & Pumariega, 2005; Rothe & Pumariega, 2012). Moreover, some authors argued that mental health care is not among the primary needs of refugees, and considerable debate exists in terms of what a refugee needs and how to provide these services (Summerfield, 1995, 2000, 2003), so the mental health needs of refugees are a source of ongoing controversy in which a knowledge base is still being developed.

This chapter presents an overview of the current numbers of refugees around the world; the types of mental health issues that affect them; the diagnosis, treatment, and systems of care that have been utilized to treat these refugees in Europe and the United States; and the risk factors and protective factors that may influence the mental health outcomes in this population.

THE CURRENT REFUGEE PROBLEM AROUND THE WORLD

Civilian populations are very often the victims of war, violence, and persecution. The number of refugees around the world is constantly changing, and developing countries were host to four fifths of the world's refugees. By the end of 2016, there were 65.6 million individuals forcibly displaced worldwide as a result of persecution, conflict, violence, or human rights violations. That was an increase of 300,000 people over the previous year, and the world's forcibly displaced population remained at a record high.

During the year 2016, there were 10.3 million people newly displaced by conflict or persecution. This included 6.9 million individuals displaced within the borders of their own countries and 3.4 million new refugees and new asylum seekers. The number of new displacements was equivalent to 20 people being forced to flee their homes every minute. Children below 18 years of age constituted about half of the refugee population in 2016, as in recent years. Children make up an estimated 31% of the total world population, and the UNHCR estimated that at least 10 million people were stateless or at risk of statelessness in 2016. However, the data captured by governments and reported to UNHCR were limited to 3.2 million stateless individuals in 75 countries, so the true total numbers are estimated to be higher.

Developing regions hosted 84% of the world's refugees. The least developed countries provided asylum to a growing proportion, with 28% of the global total (4.9 million refugees). Refugees who returned to their countries of origin increased from recent years. During 2016, there were 552,200 refugees who returned to their countries of origin, often in less-than-ideal conditions. The number is more than double than the previous year, and most of these refugees returned to Afghanistan (384,000). The number of new asylum claims around the world remained high at 2.0 million, and Germany was the world's largest recipient of new individual applications, with 722,400 such claims, followed by the United States of America (262,000), Italy (123,000), and Turkey (78,600). Lebanon continued to host the largest number of refugees relative to its national population, with 1 in 6 people a refugee. Jordan (1 in 11) and Turkey (1 in 28) ranked second and third, respectively.

More than half (55%) of all refugees worldwide came from just three countries: The Syrian Arab Republic (5.5 million), Afghanistan (2.5 million) and South Sudan (1.4 million). In 2016, the UNHCR referred 162,600 refugees to other countries for resettlement. According to government statistics, 37 countries admitted 189,300 refugees for resettlement during the year, including those resettled with UNHCR's assistance. The United States of America admitted the highest number (96,900). Unaccompanied or separated children, mainly Afghans and Syrians, lodged some 75,000 asylum applications in 70 countries during the year, although this figure is assumed to be an underestimate. Germany received the highest number of these applications (35,900) (UNHCR, 2016).

EXPLANATIONS FOR FORCED MIGRATIONS

Refugees rarely have a choice in the decision to migrate; the most common cause of sudden flight is the targeting of an individual or a group due to their tribal, racial, religious, political, or ideological identity. This may result in their actual expulsion or, more often the decision to escape is due to an attempt to avoid being arrested, segregated, tortured, or killed, sometimes in genocidal campaigns known as *ethnic cleansing*. Sometimes, people are caught in the crossfire of wars and other conflicts that have little to do with who they are, and these individuals also seek safer havens in other lands (Rose, 2014).

In the 1960s, refugees were primarily produced by decolonization, revolutions and proxy wars between the United States and the Soviet Union, and this progressed into the mid-twentieth century. The global dynamics of forced migration changed in 1991 with the end of the Cold War. Instead of conflict between states, the underlying cause of most forced migration is now ethnic or religious conflict in fragile, failing, or failed states (Keely, 1996; Nurussaman, 2009). Currently, three quarters of the world's refugees were to be found in nations neighboring their countries of origin, with more than half (55%) of all refugees worldwide coming from five countries: Afghanistan, Somalia, Iraq, Syria, and Sudan (UNHCR 2016). The case of Afghanistan is very important for debates about the causes of forced migration and its solutions. At its peak in the late 1990s, estimates suggested that about 8 million people (one to two thirds, or 64%) of all living Afghans have been refugees at one point in their lives (Rose, 2014).

PHASES OF THE REFUGEE EXPERIENCE

Refugees, especially children and adolescents, may demonstrate great resiliency in the face of adversity, yet prior to arriving in the receiving country, these refugees may undergo a series of very stressful experiences that may place them at risk for psychological distress and the development of psychiatric disorders (Rousseau, 1995). These experiences fit within the three phases of the refugees experience described next: preflight, flight, and resettlement (Lustig, Kia-Keating, Knight, et al., 2004).

Preflight

The preflight phase refers to the time before the escape from the country of origin. Refugees face social upheaval and increasing chaos. Daily routines are disrupted, and there is limited access to work. In the case of children, schools close, going outside the house becomes unsafe, and this results in a disruption of education and social development. Refugees often face threats to their safety, and many of them witness or engage in violence. Separation from relatives, parents, and caregivers is common. A study in Mozambique found that 77% of the 500 children surveyed had witnessed murders or mass killings (Boothby, 1994). In a sample of Cambodian adolescents who survived the Pol Pot regime, 98% endured forced labor, and 83% lacked sufficient food for long periods of time (Kinzie, Sack, Angell, Manson, & Rath, 1986).

Flight

During the period of flight, refugees must survive displacement from their home environments and are often at the mercy of external circumstances that they cannot control. Children's ability to self-regulate depends in large part on the availability and the emotional state of their caretakers. One of the most common effects of war and persecution on the family is the separation of family members from each other and children from caretakers. Many young refugees lack identifiable guardians and may have travelled long distances and experienced many traumatic events without adult supervision. Political violence may sometimes render entire villages devoid of adults (Lustig, Kia-Keating, Knight, et al., 2004).

In a clinic sample of 300 Cuban child and adolescent refugees seen in an infirmary located inside a refugee camp, 58% of preschool-age and 31% of school-age children had been separated from their fathers during the process of flight (Rothe, 2005). In another sample of 100 Cuban adolescents released from refugee camps and seen after arrival in the United States, 69% had left behind grandparents, and 79% had left behind aunts, uncles, and other members of their extended families, many of whom were the child's primary caretakers while the parents worked (Rothe, Castillo-Matos, & Busquets, 2002).

Many refugee children and adolescents enter the United States as undocumented aliens and later seek asylum, while others come from refugee camps, usually situated on foreign soil. In these camps, inhabitants are depersonalized, becoming numbers without names, and traumatic events are common. In a study of Cuban children and adolescents who left the island on rafts and boats and were later detained in refugee camps prior to arriving in the United States, the refugees reported that during their ocean crossing they faced storms at sea that caused their sea crafts to capsize, they witnessed people drown, and they observed floating corpses being devoured by sharks. Once in the refugee camps, 80% of these children and adolescents witnessed acts of violence, and 37% saw someone attempt or commit suicide (Rothe, Castillo-Matos, et al., 2002; Rothe, Lewis, et al., 2002). While they were interned in the refugee camps, many of these children and adolescents experienced soiling, bedwetting, and nightmares and exhibited aggressive behavior, separation anxiety, and other regressive behaviors (Rothe, 2005).

Children who come to the United States without a guardian must negotiate the legal system without advocates. Children awaiting asylum hearings in the United States are sometimes held up to 2 years in detention facilities or juvenile jails. Resources for refugee children are scarce, and many who may have legitimate asylum claims are unaware of their legal rights (Rothe & Pumariega, 2012).

Resettlement

The loss of the homeland, family, friends, and material possessions characterizes the resettlement stage. Once refugees resettle in the new host country, they need to undergo a process of acculturation, which brings about inherent stressors (Rousseau, 1995). Refugees and families often need to learn a new language and have to adjust to new values, beliefs systems, social mores, and family roles, which causes stress to all the members of the family. In the process of resettlement and acculturation, refugees often undergo stages similar to the type of profound mourning process that follows a massive personal loss (Rothe, Tzuang, & Pumariega, 2010).

Continued psychological distress in this stage may result from delays in processing asylum applications, uncertainty about asylum status, negotiation with immigration authorities, obstacles with employment, inadequate housing, frequent moves, language problems, racial discrimination, and social isolation (De Antiss et al., 2009; Ehntholt & Yule, 2006). For example, unfavorable living conditions, such as living in communal shelters, have been found to increase psychological stress in war-exposed children (Ajdukovic & Ajdukovic, 1993).

UNACCOMPANIED CHILD AND ADOLESCENT REFUGEES

Unaccompanied child refugees typically flee their nations alone to avoid threats of persecution or violence toward them or their families, threat of war and resulting victimization, threat of recruitment as child soldiers or enslavement, or after the death of parents or guardians during war or political strife (Ehntholt & Yule, 2006). They are typically exposed to a higher number of traumatic stressors prior to fleeing than their accompanied counterparts. For example, in one study (Thomas, Thomas, Nafees, & Bhugra, 2004), 32% of unaccompanied child refugees reported having been raped, including some males.

They are at greater vulnerability to traumas not only in their home nation that prompted escape, but also during their stays in refugee camps and during the initial period of resettlement in host nations. The last can include placement in group homes or foster homes with little supervision or support, victimization at the hands of caregivers or peers, as well as their isolation as a result of their separation or loss of their natural families. Uncertain legal status can also complicate their emotional adjustment and contribute to their being further isolated in detention facilities in host nations for extended periods, interfering with their resettlement adjustment and acculturation process.

Unaccompanied child refugees have been shown to have higher levels of symptoms of psychological distress than their accompanied counterparts (Fox, Cowell, & Montgomery, 1994; McKelvey & Webb, 1995; Sourander, 1998). They may also encounter ambivalence and even ostracism and rejection by their natural family at the time of reunification as a result of their psychological/mental health problems, which can have repercussions on the family as well. Their distress may also not be believed and validated by their natural families at the time of reunification, in part out of denial and guilt by their parents at having made the decision to allow them to emigrate alone.

CHILD SOLDIERS

There are approximately 300,000 child soldiers under 18 years of age actively fighting in 14 different countries around the world today. Child soldiers are at risk of exposure to rape, torture, and war injuries and may later suffer from substance abuse, depression, and anxiety. In addition, child soldiers lose trust in authority figures and also may lose their moral perspective, engaging in stealing, looting, and killing, while being ordered to do so and told that killing for political reasons is morally justified. The complexity of psychodynamic factors involved in being a child soldier often translates into feelings in which the military becomes a surrogate family, particularly in children separated from their biological families. There is a scarcity of information regarding the long-term mental health outcomes and efforts at reintegration into society of these child soldiers, including where they end up seeking asylum and what happens in their lives when they become adults, given that many chose to remain silent about their past experiences (Human Rights Watch, 2018; Lustig, Kia-Keating, Knight, et al., 2004; Schnauer & Elbert, 2010).

EPIDEMIOLOGICAL FINDINGS

The literature does not provide consistent prevalence rates for psychiatric disorders in refugees, owing mostly to differences in samples, methods, and instrumentation. Also, there is wide variability in the exposure to different forms of trauma (De Antiss et al., 2009). There is agreement among investigators that PTSD is higher among refugees and asylum seekers than in the general population, with studies reporting between 3% and 86%. One meta-analysis described the rate of mental health conditions as twice as high among refugees and asylum seekers compared to those who migrated for economic reasons (Lindert, Ehrenstein, Priebe, Mielck, & Brahler, 2009).

In their systematic review of 20 surveys with 6,743 refugees (260 were children), Fazel, Wheeler, and Danesh (2005) found an overall rate of PTSD of 11%. McKelvey and colleagues (2002) found a prevalence rate of 18% among refugee children residing in Australia, with this rate lower than a previous Australian report of 32% (Krupinski & Burrows, 1986). Studies in the United States focusing on the effects of extreme trauma on refugee children calculated the rates of psychiatric disorders at 40%–50% (Kinzie, Sack, Angell, & Clarke, 1989; Kinzie et al., 1986; Sack, Him, & Dickason, 1999), very similar to the rates estimated in Britain (Hodes, 1998).

Various authors reported that the prevalence rates of mental health disorders and physical health problems among refugees increased in proportion to the length of the asylum procedure, while their life satisfaction decreased accordingly (Laban, Gernaat, Komproe, & De Jong, 2007; Laban, Gernaat, Komproe, Schreuders, & De Jong, 2004; Laban, Gernaat, Komproe, Van Tweel, & De Jong, 2005). Because certain factors are known to increase PTSD, this may also help explain the wide variations between studies. Nevertheless, there seems to be agreement that refugee children and adults are at a higher risk of developing multiple, coexisting psychiatric disorders than the general population, and this risk is calculated in some studies to be as high as 30.6% (Aichenberger, 2015) and in other studies as high as 40% (Hodes, 2000).

SOME CONTROVERSIES IN DEFINING THE REFUGEE EXPERIENCE ACROSS CULTURES

The refugee mental health literature reveals a problem-centered research agenda, with most research focused on the diagnosis, treatment, and prognosis of PTSD, which is believed to result from the refugee experience (De Antiss et al., 2009; Ehntholt & Yule, 2006; Lurie & Nakash, 2015; Ozkan & Belz, 2015). Opponents state that it is wrong to apply a Western biomedical classification to diverse cultures on the basis that refugees are responding normally to abnormal situations. The use of psychiatric labeling has been criticized as a form of stigmatization, which fails to take into account the losses and adversities of refugees and to account for the context of their human condition (Baarnhielm & Mosko, 2015; Kuey, 2015; Lurie & Nakash, 2015; Ozkan & Belz, 2015; Summerfield, 2000; Westermeyer & Janca, 1997).

This controversy is tied to a more philosophical debate about the legitimacy and existence of mental illness. The "positivist" movement acknowledges the existence of mental illness across cultures, whereas the "constructionist" movement argues that mental illness is specific to the particular cultural context and cannot exist legitimately as a universal concept (Silove, 2005). The movement also indicates that there are significant variations in the manifestations and treatment of mental illness across cultures, and that it is inappropriate and unwise to apply Western psychiatric models without first understanding the cultural context in which these phenomena take place (Baarnhielm & Mosko, 2015; Kleinman, 1987). A third viewpoint argues that even though there may be substantial variability across cultures in terms of the expression symptoms and prevalence rates, these controversies can be resolved if future studies can be more rigorous in their methodology, with the use of culturally validated research instruments, bilingual interviewers, random samples, and control groups (Minas & Sawyer, 2002; Porter & Haslam, 2005; Silove, 1999).

This debate serves to highlight the complexity of the bio-psycho-social issues involved in the refugee experience. Other authors argued that even though many emotional reactions are expectable given the circumstances faced by refugees, they still require treatment interventions to alleviate the child's psychological distress, and that diagnosing and labeling may be a useful way to mobilize resources to provide the needed help. In addition, they argued that PTSD can be understood as a neurophysiological disorder characterized by an exaggerated response to the fight–flight reaction, with the only differences presenting themselves in the cultural expressions of distress (Ehntholt & Yule, 2006; Hodes, 2002). Developmental theory is also essential to understanding the experience of refugee children and adolescents. Experiences of war and persecution may result in feelings of mistrust, betrayal, humiliation, and a sense of vulnerability in children and adolescents, who depend on adults for guidance and safety. If the child's trust in the adult's ability to care for them is shaken, this may complicate or derail the stages of their normal psychological development (Lustig, Kia-Keating, Knight, et al., 2004).

However, assumptions about development, normality, and psychopathology are culturally embedded, and some authors have criticized their reliance on Western values and their generalizability to other populations. They argued that this approach may exaggerate psychiatric pathology in refugees and lead to an increase in mental health service utilization while downplaying their resiliency and strengths (Rechtman, 2000; Summerfield, 1999, 2000; Watters, 2001; Zarowsky, 2000).

Some health models integrate culture and psychological development, in particular ecological systems theory (Brofenbrenner, 1979), which explains that human beings develop in an interaction with their environment that takes place at four levels: the macrosystem (societal rules and beliefs); exosystem (community and neighborhood factors); microsystem (the family); and the ontogenic level (individual factors). The interplay between these four levels explains how the impact of culture, economics, family support systems, and individual strengths or vulnerabilities may ultimately affect the adaptation and overall well-being of the refugees. This model is also useful in designing treatment interventions that are acceptable and appropriate to the particular individual and the individual's family (Hodes, 2002), including their cultural views of traumatic events, life cycles, and family systems (Lustig, Kia-Keating, Knight, et al., 2004; Pumariega, Rothe, & Pumariega, 2005; Tseng, 2001).

A new way of thinking about the refugee problem worldwide is to conceptualize the trauma produced by forced migrations as a global challenge. The challenge has three parts. The first is to examine the effects of international violence and wars with the social systems from which they originate. Second, there is a need to take into account that trauma-related conditions will present with various cultural idioms of distress that need to be incorporated in the treatment designs for these populations. The third acknowledges that it is fundamental to integrate psycho-social and biological approaches to better understand the causality and, in turn, to design more effective treatments for these populations (Pedersen, 2015).

MENTAL HEALTH DIFFICULTIES IN REFUGEES

A review of 29 studies involving 16,010 refugees of war found (1) high prevalence rates of depression, PTSD, and other anxiety disorders among refugees 5 years or longer after displacement, with prevalence estimates typically in the range of 20% and above; and (2) a number of unique risk factors for mental disorders that included higher exposure to traumatic experiences, and postmigration stress, such as poor postmigration socioeconomic situation (unemployment, low income, poor host language proficiency, and lack of social support), was associated with depression, and being a female refugee was associated with higher levels of anxiety but not PTSD (Bogic, Njoku, & Priebe, 2015). Other findings included that the risk of having a serious mental disorder was substantially (14 times) higher in war refugees than in the general population, even several years after refugee resettlement, and the risk of developing PTSD was 15 times higher than in the general population. In the case of child and adolescent refugees, many have been exposed to experiences of persecution, violence, war, killing, or torture as well as the subsequent losses, which increase the risk of psychological distress and psychiatric disorders. PTSD symptoms have been found in children exposed to persecution, war, and organized violence in many parts of the world, including Cambodia (Sack, Seeley, & Clarke, 1997); Rwanda (Dyregrov, Gupta, Gjestad, & Mukanoheli, 2000); Kuwait (Nader, Pynoos, Fairbanks, Al-Ajeel, & Al-Asfour, 1993); Palestine (Thabet & Vostanis, 1999); Afghanistan (Mghir, Freed, Raskin, & Katon, 1995); Bosnia (Papageorgiou et al., 2000); and Cuba (Rothe, 2005).

Depression, anxiety, and grief are also commonly found among refugees. However, the estimates of coexisting psychiatric disorders vary widely depending on the type of events experienced, the population studied, and the diagnostic methods that are employed. For example, anxiety was reported among 4%–8% Vietnamese (Felsman, Leong, Johnson, & Felsman, 1990); 11.5% of Tibetan (Servan-Schreiber, Le Lin, & Birmaher, 1998); and 47% of Bosnian (Papageorgiou et al., 2000) child and adolescent refugees. Depression commonly coexists with PTSD and anxiety. For example, in a group of 59 Cambodian refugee adolescent and young adults exposed to trauma as children, 24% had PTSD, while 57% had an additional affective or anxiety disorder, with major depression and generalized anxiety disorder the most common (Kinzie et al., 1986; Sack et al., 1994).

Although grief reactions are also common among refugees, these have rarely been investigated. In a sample of 8- to 21-year-old Kuwaiti refugees following the Gulf War, 98% reported at least one symptom of grief (Nader et al., 1993), and similar levels of grief were reported among Bosnian children exposed to war (Smith, Perrin, Yule, Hacam, & Stuvland, 2002). Shannon, Weiling, Simmelink-McCleary, and Becher (2015) explored the effects of political trauma and torture in 111 adult refugees who arrived in the United States from Bhutan, Burma, Ethiopia, and Somalia. These refugees reported (1) experiencing mental distress, defined as "craziness" in each of their native languages; (2) "too much thinking"; (3) cognitive effects such as memory loss, confusion, and difficulty with concentration; (4) physical symptoms such as headaches, stomachaches, and palpitations; (5) behavioral effects, such as abuse of substances, irritability, startle reactions, inability to sleep, talking too much or being at a loss for words, avoidance, and suicidal ideation; and (6) emotional sensations and reactions such as fear, anger, sadness, depression, shame, guilt, frustration, hopelessness, and helplessness over past traumatic events, which was described as "burning emotionality." Other commonly reported, but less well-researched, problems that affect younger refugees include physical complaints, sleep problems, social problems, conduct disorder, social withdrawal, attention problems, generalized fear, overdependency, restlessness, irritability, and difficulties in peer relationships (Mollica, Poole, Son, & Murray, 1997; Rothe, 2005; Rothe, Castillo, et al., 1998; Tousignant et al., 1999); learning difficulties and problems with school functioning (Rousseau, Drapeau, & Corin, 1996); defiance, hyperactivity, and aggression (Hjern, Angel, & Hojer, 1991; Rothe, Castillo-Matos, Brinson, & Lewis, 2000); and eating disorders (Fahy, Robinson, Russell, & Sheinman, 1988). Among child refugees, there can be a loss of previously acquired skills, such as loss of bladder control with secondary bedwetting, soiling, intense separation anxiety, and nail-biting (Chimienti, Nasr, & Khalifeh, 1989; Rothe, Castillo-Matos, et al., 2000). Sadness, introversion, and tiredness (Ehntholt, 2005); suicidal ideation and attempted suicide (Bodegard, 2005; Tousignant et al., 1999); and violent self-harm (Patel & Hodes, 2006) have also been reported. The risk for developing psychosis has been found to be increased in adolescent refugees (Tolmac & Hodes, 2004). A syndrome of pervasive devitalization has been described in young asylum seekers, characterized by a refusal to eat, drink, talk, walk, engage socially, or accept help (Bodegard, 2005; von Folsach & Montgomery, 2006).

Young refugees also present problems that would have developed even if they had not been exposed to war or persecution, such as attention deficit hyperactivity disorder, learning disabilities, developmental disorders

(Howard & Hodes, 2000; Rothe, 2005; Williams & Westermeyer, 1983), asthma, and epilepsy (Rothe, 2005), and these may be exacerbated by migration. It is important to note that the presence of PTSD appears to be related to earlier experiences of war trauma and resettlement stress, while depression tends to exacerbate after arrival in the receiving country and is linked to recent life difficulties and acculturation stress, such as poor spoken English (Sack, Clarke, & Seeley, 1996).

PROTECTIVE FACTORS

Refugee resiliency has been poorly studied but is beginning to receive more attention. Studies of adult refugees conclude that effective social integration into the host country is associated with better mental health in men, but not in women. Women and girls are more prone to having been victims of sexual violence during war and inside the refugee camps (Abraham, Lien, & Hanssen, 2018). Endless waiting and uncertainty about the future while in refugee camps worsens mental health issues of refugees and leads to a sense of helplessness and catastrophic thinking (Abraham et al., 2018; Rothe, 2005, 2008).

In contrast, thinking about the future, with dreams of furthering their education, resuming a normal life and reuniting with loved ones improved coping. Many refugees experienced great joy when reencountering peers and loved ones and reestablishing past relationships. The concept of "having someone to share one's thoughts with," especially someone who had shared the same experiences, was found to be very healing. The concept of a person's *sense of coherence*, which derives from the field of positive psychology, postulates that individuals who feel empowered to make change in their lives and surroundings and see life as comprehensible, manageable, and meaningful and not as life events that are inevitable with the person at the mercy of their fate have better mental health outcomes (Seligman & Csikszentmihalyi, 2000). This perspective allows the refugee to think positively, learn, and grow from the experiences (Rothe, 2005; Rothe, Castillo-Matos, et al., 2002).

The role of religion has also been found to foster resiliency in refugees. Having faith in God and in God's plan for the person's future, counting on the support from a religious community, being grateful for having survived, trusting that future difficulties will be overcome with God's help, and the soothing effects of prayer, meditation, and spirituality have been found to be helpful when facing difficult circumstances. Also, the sense of collectivism, of feeling part of a community, including experiencing feelings of empathy, dependency, and reciprocity toward other members of the group and having a sense of belonging, are important in resiliency (Abraham et al., 2018; Steel, Silove, Phan, & Bauman, 2002).

Many refugee children have been found to be free of mental health problems (Hodes, 2000; Summerfield, 2000), while others cope quite well (Mollica et al., 1997; Rothe, Lewis, et al., 2002; Sack et al., 1999; Tousignant et al., 1999), and many show improvement over time (Almqvist & Broberg, 1999; Almqvist & Brandell-Forsberg, 1997; Hjern & Angel, 2000). Some of the factors that contribute to resiliency in young refugees include being of a young age at the time of the trauma, having good self-esteem, having a temperament that allows responding well and effectively to new situations, having religious faith (Almqvist & Broberg, 1999; Garmezy & Rutter, 1985), and having strong ideological commitment to their side of the cause (Punamäki, 1996; Servan-Schreiber et al., 1998). Adaptability and cohesion within families, positive psychological well-being of caregivers, and good peer group and social supports have been found to be protective during the refugee process as well as during the resettlement period (Ajdukovic & Ajdukovic, 1993; Almqvist & Broberg, 1999; Rousseau & Drapeau, 2003). A meta-analysis of refugee mental health research found that children may be less symptomatic, have better psycho-social functioning, and be more resilient than adults (Porter & Haslam, 2005).

LONG-TERM PROGNOSIS

Psychiatric symptoms and mental health difficulties of refugees have been found to persist over many years. A small study of Cambodian children exposed to massive trauma found that, 4 years after leaving Cambodia, 50% met diagnostic criteria for PTSD and 53% for depression (Kinzie et al., 1986). Depressive symptoms tended to decrease over time, but later increased again after 12 years (Kinzie et al., 1986; Sack et al., 1993, 1999). However, certain investigators have cautioned that these studies described children who suffered extreme trauma and privations, and that the rates of recovery could be slower than in other, less traumatized samples (Ehntholt & Yule, 2006). A different study with Iranian preschool refugee children found that symptoms decreased over a period of 2½ years, but that after that period of time, 82% still had symptoms, and 21% met diagnostic criteria for PTSD (Almqvist & Brandell-Forsberg, 1997). A study of Cuban adolescent refugees attending schools in the United States after their release from refugee camps revealed that self-report measures of post-traumatic symptoms were elevated, yet the teachers in charge of the students were unable to detect any symptoms when rating these students with a standardized questionnaire (Rothe, Lewis, et al., 2002).

These and other studies revealed that sometimes child and adolescent refugees experience their symptoms silently, while other responsible adults, such as teachers or parents, are unable to detect their distress. The available research suggests that a long time after the events took place, many young refugees continue to suffer from distressing symptoms, especially those of PTSD. Despite these symptoms, considerable amount of research indicates that most people exposed to trauma recover naturally over time and do not report significant psychopathology (Rothbaum, Foa, Riggs, Murdock, & Walsh, 1992). Refugees, especially young refugees, also tend to function relatively well overall, both socially and academically (Kinzie et al., 1989; Rothe, Lewis, et al., 2002).

MENTAL HEALTH ASSESSMENT AND SCREENING OF REFUGEES

The federal Refugee Act of 1980 entitles newly arrived refugees to a comprehensive health assessment and referral to health services and assistance or state Medicaid in their first 8 months. This makes it even more imperative that screening and referral for assessment and treatment take place early in the resettlement process. There is also a growing body of literature that indicates that refugees struggle with substance use, and families may be vulnerable to domestic violence both in camps and after they are resettled. A national survey on refugees who had been victims of torture (Shannon et al., 2012) revealed that only half of the states provided any mental health screening to newly arrived refugees. Of the states that provide screening for mental health symptoms, more than half utilize informal conversation. Further, less than half the states reported directly asking refugees about their exposure to war trauma or torture.

The most frequently cited reasons for not providing mental health screening were the lack of culturally sensitive instruments and the lack of time and resources. For adult refugees, there have been various attempts at adapting the Harvard Trauma Questionnaire to diverse ethnic populations (Hollifield et al., 2002). In the case of children and adolescents, a number of instruments have been identified, but very few have been used extensively with refugees. The majority of the diagnostic instruments have been designed and validated for Western, Caucasian, mainstream, majority populations in developed countries and may not be valid when used with peoples of other cultures. In addition, most diagnostic instruments have been designed to overidentify pathology, so the data must be interpreted with extreme caution.

Kinzie and colleagues (2006) are of the opinion that it is not appropriate to use standardized questionnaires with child and adolescent refugees, only extensive, open-ended interviewing and assessment, in order to establish a diagnosis. Ehntholt and Yule (2006), based on their experience in Britain, have designed a semistructured interview for assessing child and adolescent refugees. They recommended that only when the diagnosis is not clear, or when writing legal reports, should standardized questionnaires be used. Birman and Chan (2008) have developed parameters to assess child and adolescent refugees in schools. They highlighted that universal mental health screening of refugee children in schools is not advised given that it may unnecessarily label and stigmatize children and may also identify more problems than the school or community can treat. They also enumerated other barriers that interfere with universal mental health screening, such as obtaining informed consent from parents and other sociocultural issues. Many of the parents may speak a language for which there are few available interpreters and sometimes may not even be literate in their own language. Sometimes, parents may assume that if they are being called by the school, it is because the child "is in trouble and needs to be punished."

Because refugee families are dealing with a multitude of stressors, a "team approach" is the most feasible as well as a model of co-joint consultation, which includes involving prominent members of the refugee community, many of whom may themselves be former refugees or immigrants, as well as refugee and community agencies or religious institutions. A comprehensive list and description of the standardized mental health assessment questionnaires for child and adolescent refugees can be found in the work of Birman and Chan (2008) and Ehntholt and Yule (2006).

TREATMENT INTERVENTIONS AND SERVICES: ACCESS TO CARE

Traditional Western mental health services and treatment approaches have not been historically effective with immigrants and refugees. They often underutilize traditional mental health services as a result of numerous internal and external barriers. These include the stigma associated with mental illness and treatment in their cultures and countries of origin (usually stronger than that seen in Western nations); a lack of clinicians who speak the languages and understand the cultures of refugees; low priority for obtaining mental health services among more pressing human needs (food, shelter, employment, etc.); and lack of finances or insurance coverage to pay for services (Ehntholt & Yule, 2006). The principles of culturally competent mental health services and community-based systems of care are most applicable to the development and delivery of mental health services for refugees (Pumariega, Rogers, & Rothe, 2005;

Pumariega, Rothe, & Rogers, 2009; Pumariega et al., 2013). These include accounting for cultural differences that can impact diagnostic assessment; addressing factors that affect the accessibility and acceptability (e.g., location, stigma, linguistic barriers, documentation, and legal status); addressing traumatic and acculturation themes in psychotherapy; empowerment, psychoeducation, and collaboration with families); and integrating traditional mental health services with primary care services and natural community supports from the immigrant or refugee community (including collaboration with spiritual resources and cultural healers).

For example, Vietnamese immigrants with mental illness have been found to use local Vietnamese-speaking physicians, Asian naturalists, spiritual and folk healers, as well as psychiatric facilities and community mental health services (Phan, 2000). Russian immigrants, on the other hand, tend to use individual outpatient services at voluntary nonprofit agencies (Chow, Jaffee, & Choi, 1999). Mexican immigrants, on the other hand, prefer primary care physicians to formal mental health services (Pumariega, Glover, Holzer, & Nguyen, 1998). Cultural consultants with knowledge of the immigrant and refugee communities have been found to be particularly effective in facilitating accurate assessment and improved services utilization and effectiveness (Kirmayer, Groleau, Guzder, Blake, & Jarvis, 2003). Approaches that address the need for validation, mutual support, and processing of their common migration and adaptation experiences have been found to be particularly effective (Dossa, 2002; Simich, Beiser, & Mawani, 2003).

In dealing with refugee crises, sometimes the receiving community may find itself besieged by a massive arrival of refugees, which may overwhelm the available mental health infrastructure. To avoid this situation, it is advisable to compose teams of mental health professionals that take into account the particular circumstances of the refugee crisis and the particular cultural and language characteristics of the of the refugee group in question. Culturally competent professionals must compose the treatment groups and, if they are not proficient in the particular language of the members of the refugee group, translator services should then become indispensable (Sack et al., 1997).

Treatment interventions should start at the level of refugee groups within camps, following the similar parameters of those of victims of natural disasters and can be divided into three phases: triage, debriefing, and emergency services. The first intervention involves triaging the most psychologically severely affected refugees (the "psychological casualties") in order to provide the immediate necessary treatment interventions to the victims. Child refugees and their families often suffer cognitive disorganization as a result of the multiple stresses to which they have been subjected and that result from the process of traumatic migrations. The process of debriefing aims to validate the traumatic and disorganizing quality of the experience and to inform and orient the refugees about their new surrounding reality. The traumatic events and their associated emotional, behavioral, and physical reactions are revisited, analyzed, and understood in the context of the surrounding circumstances. Activities are designed in order to provide structure, help organize time, and plan daily activities, including work activities, in an attempt to normalize routines. This prevents the child and the family's cognitive disorganization and its consequences. Supporting indigenous religious practices and culturally prescribed altruistic practices among refugees also supports resiliency and recovery (Mollica, Cui, McInnes, & Massagli, 2002; Rothe, Castillo-Matos, et al., 2002). Rothe (2008) has developed a psychotherapy model for treating child and adolescent refugees living inside refugee camps in order to minimize psychological trauma and to prevent dissociative memories that result from these experiences.

TREATMENT PROCESS

Most of the treatments for adult and child refugees have been designed utilizing the model of PTSD; however, literature relating to the treatment of PTSD in refugees has been described and has been shown to be limited by methodological difficulties, including nonrandom allocation to treatment, lack of controls, and nonblind outcome assessments. In a review of the psychological therapies for treatment of PTSD in adult refugees, Nicholli and Thompson (2004) concluded the following:

1. The presentation and validity construct of PTSD is open to debate due to cultural and linguistic factors.
2. The nature of trauma experienced by refugees may differ from typically occurring Western traumas and as such may be novel for clinicians.
3. Multiple, extremely severe, and prolonged traumatic incidents may be common and require complex treatment approaches.
4. The use of standard assessment measures can be criticized as lacking in reliability and validity with this population.
5. Efficacious PTSD psychotherapeutic treatment approaches have been developed and evaluated within Western countries, and as such the findings of these will not necessarily generalize to other cultures.
6. The use of an interpreter removes the traditional therapeutic dyad and may slow the pace of therapy. Also, listening to trauma stories and the distress of clients is potentially overwhelming and may impact both therapists and interpreters.
7. Refugees are often undergoing additional life stresses (poverty, loss of status, uncertainty of residence, discrimination, and prejudice), which raises the question of when or even whether to address psychological issues in the presence of pressing fundamental needs.
8. Clinicians will be faced with exploring cultural and religious practices that are likely to be different from their own and may stimulate strong countertransference feelings and possibly underlying prejudices.

In a more recent study, Small et al. (2016) compared (1) office-based counseling, (2) home-based counseling, and (3) community-based psychoeducational group treatment to treat post-traumatic stress symptoms, depression, anxiety, and somatization and to provide social support for adult resettled refugees of various nationalities. They found all interventions were relatively effective. In addition, they discovered that using a practical and yet less threatening mental health intervention facilitated by community leaders and counselors can also have positive effects on serious mental health problems and should be studied further.

Testimonial psychotherapy in adults has also yielded promising results (Weine, Kulenovic, Dzubur, Pavkovic, & Gibbons, 1998). In the work with refugee children and adolescents, a phased specific model approach is important because the children may still be undergoing significant turmoil in their lives. Movement back and forth between phases is common. This is especially true for children and families seeking asylum, for whom emotional states are heavily influenced by changes in asylum status and the impact these have on life circumstances (Ehntholt & Yule, 2006). The three main phases to be considered are (1) establishment of safety and trust; (2) trauma-focused therapy/treatment; and (3) reintegration.

The aims during the stage of establishment of safety and trust are to help the child and family develop a sense of stability, safety, and trust, as well as to regain a sense of control over their lives. This may be difficult to achieve until stable asylum status is granted, so clinicians must have an awareness of immigration law, welfare rights, and the sociopolitical situation in the home nation. Liaison work with agencies is necessary in order to ensure that basic needs and supports are addressed. Initial sessions may need to focus on solving housing and financial problems, as well as facilitating access to reputable attorneys, family tracing services, and educational, health, religious, cultural, and leisure resources. Psychoeducation regarding symptoms and treatment models, normalizing reactions to trauma, and symptom management and coping strategies are key interventions, with trauma work not advisable due to the family and child's state of continued vulnerability. They are ready for the next stage only after the child and family feel some sense of safety and stability, control over their symptoms, and some level of trust.

For children suffering from symptoms of PTSD, the trauma-focused therapy/treatment phase involves working through traumatic events (at a pace that is emotionally manageable) to create a coherent and detailed narrative of past experiences that is more integrated into their life story. This should include the exploration of feelings of guilt and shame from witnessing violence or murder, reframing them within the context of political and developmental realities and issues of loss and bereavement. The therapist bears witness and validates the traumatic experiences that the child has experienced. Depending on the young person's current complaints, alternative interventions may be offered at this stage for a range of difficulties, including depression, anxiety, sleep problems, somatic complaints, and behavioral difficulties.

The focus during reintegration is on creating future goals and aspirations and integrating into a new community and culture. Young refugees will have already begun this process on their own, with help from schools and community resources. The therapist could discuss educational plans, geographic relocation, or future employment with refugee children and families to help develop a pathway toward these goals. Child refugees and their families can also become more involved in their religious or immigrant communities or in school extracurricular and social activities.

TREATMENT MODALITIES AND PREVENTIVE INTERVENTIONS

Evidence-based treatments for many conditions, including those affecting refugees, are now available. However, it is a challenge to provide these in catastrophic situations, such as refugee camps, underserved areas, and rural areas. Bolton et al. (2014) tested the Common Elements Treatment Approach (CETA) with Burmese refugees living in Thailand. This approach trains nonprofessional counselors to apply some necessary elements of evidence-based treatments to treat refugees residing in low-income settings who suffer from depression, anxiety, and post-traumatic stress. In a randomized controlled study, they found that there was a 77% reduction in the average depression score from before the intervention to after the intervention among participants in the CETA arm, but only a 40% reduction in the depression score among participants in the control arm.

Different models of types of psychotherapy have been found effective in addressing the mental health needs of refugee children and their families (Ehntholt & Yule, 2006). Trauma-focused cognitive behavioral therapy (CBT) has demonstrated effectiveness with diverse populations and even has a track record with child refugee populations. A controlled study of group CBT with refugee children from various nations demonstrated that it was effective at reducing PTSD symptoms, as well as behavioral difficulties and emotional symptoms resulting from war-related trauma (Ehntholt, Smith, & Yule, 2005).

Testimonial psychotherapy invites refugees to transcend the grief, anger, and resentment resulting from their persecution by using the resulting testimonies for purposes of education and advocacy. A pilot study with Sudanese adolescents suggested its safety and feasibility in this age group (Lustig, Weine, Saxe, & Beardslee, 2004). Narrative exposure therapy combines elements of testimonial psychotherapy with cognitive behavioral techniques and theory. One of the goals of this approach is to reduce PTSD symptoms by not only confronting the individual with memories of the traumatic event, but also using a detailed narrative to correct distortion of traumatic memories. It has been recently adapted for use with refugee children and has provided reports of positive outcomes (Onyut et al., 2005).

Eye movement desensitization and reprocessing therapy (EMDR) is a treatment that uses bilateral stimulation when processing traumatic memories in individuals with PTSD. With this method, the person is often asked to conjure up an image of the traumatic event while the therapist simultaneously moves his or her finger in front of the young person's eyes in a rhythmic, lateral motion. The treatment involves a combination of both exposure and distraction or "dual attention" as it is most frequently called. A small study ($N = 13$) reported significant improvements using EMDR with refugee children experiencing PTSD symptoms (Oras, Cancela de Ezpeleta, & Ahmad, 2004).

Empirically tested interventions operating within community settings have been preliminarily promising. Kataoka et al. (2003) demonstrated the effectiveness of a school-based CBT program for trauma-related depression or post-traumatic stress with Hispanic children and youth, using group and individual CBT and psychoeducational interventions for youth and parents. Layne et al. (2001) reported on a school-based trauma- and grief-focused group psychotherapy that significantly reduced post-traumatic stress, depression, and grief symptoms among 55 war-exposed Bosnian adolescents.

Pharmacotherapy has been shown to be useful in the treatment of depression and PTSD symptoms in nonrefugee children and youth, though it was most effective in combination with CBT (Cohen and the Workgroup on Quality Issues, 2010; Curry et al., 2006). Selective serotonin reuptake inhibitors, anticonvulsants, and atypical antipsychotics have been identified as most useful, though studies with refugee children are lacking. Clonidine was shown to be effective for psychiatric symptoms among Cambodian adults with PTSD (Kinzie & Leung, 1989).

There are beginning models for preventive community-based mental health services for immigrant and refugee children and their families. Rousseau and Guzder (2008) described a number of promising school-based prevention programs for refugee children. The National Center for Mental Health Promotion and Youth Violence Prevention at Education Development Center (2011) reviews a number of promising preventive models, and practices are being implemented around the United States facilitating the adaptation of these models for immigrant and refugee children and their families; most of these models are oriented around schools.

These programs promote the development of adaptational skills by the child and develop family and community supports. They include (1) newcomer programs, 6–18 months in length, to bridge gaps in students' academic backgrounds and integrate them quickly into the regular school program. These programs also offer cross-cultural orientation and community resource orientation and connections for children and families (e.g., healthcare, mental health, social services, career counseling, tutoring, housing, and employment).

Also included are (2) programs for immigrant and limited English proficiency (LEP) parents that combine English as a second language (ESL) instruction with social support, addressing topics such as dating norms, dangers of gang involvement, and postsecondary education opportunities. They also help parents overcome language barriers and cultural understanding of the role of teachers and the public school system.

Afterschool programs (3) include activities (academic assistance, language tutoring, behavioral counseling, and recreational opportunities) that have been identified as increasingly important for helping immigrant youth improve academic achievement, stay in school, and avoid risky behaviors such as pregnancy and substance abuse. All of these models have demonstrated considerable success with a diverse range of populations, including Latino, Bosnian, Hmong, and African immigrant and refugee communities.

For unaccompanied children and adolescent refugees, group psychosocial interventions can help refugees to address such isolation and lack of validation through shared stories of their experiences, shared problem-solving, and the creation of a mutual support network (Heaphy, Ehntholt, & Sclare, 2007). However, care must be taken not to overgeneralize the findings from the limited research studies reported here. However, a key conclusion appears to be a reminder that it is particularly important for the therapist to appreciate and explore individual clients' cultural beliefs, including religious, spiritual, and ritualistic practices, as well as the individual personal beliefs and appraisals. It is important to recognize the need for greater therapist awareness and ability to work with issues of diversity and a willingness to facilitate access to appropriate practical support.

IMPLICATIONS FOR POLICY, PRACTICE, AND RESEARCH

It is very likely that the numbers of refugees worldwide will continue to increase as a result of regional warfare and conflict, so it is reasonable to expect large numbers of refugees will continue to immigrate to the United States and other developed nations seeking safety, security, and freedom

(UNHCR, 2016). Mental health and support services are most effective in the context of a refugee and immigration policy based on rational national interests rather than on reactions to crises or to xenophobia.

Part of such a policy should be to actively prepare all Americans for the demographic changes resulting in increased cultural diversity, culminating in the lack of any numerical majorities by 2050. Refugees have historically been a significant proportion of the immigrant population in the United States. Our nation should develop and implement resettlement policies and practices (in human services and education) that facilitate refugees in learning their new host culture while retaining the strength-based, adaptive aspects of their cultures of origin. The media and all institutions in civil society, including schools, churches and volunteer organizations should be recruited toward this important endeavor.

Such public education efforts can support enhanced efforts toward proactive refugee services (including mental health services), preventive cultural adaptation programs, and community supports for all immigrant children and their families. International exchange of treatment models and techniques that are effective in diverse cultures and with special populations is also particularly important in order to disseminate and build on the experience developed in the field with such models.

REFERENCES

Abraham, R., Lien, L., & Hanssen, I. (2018). Coping, resilience and posttraumatic growth among Eritrean female refugees living in Norwegian asylum reception centres: A qualitative study. *International Journal of Social Psychiatry*, *64*(4), 359–366.

Aichenberger, M. C. (2015). The epidemiology of post-traumatic stress disorder: A focus on immigrant and refugee populations (pp. 33–37). In M. Schouler-Ocak (Ed.), *Trauma and migration*. Basel, Switzerland: Springer International.

Ajdukovic, M., & Ajdukovic, D. (1993). Psychological well-being of refugee children. *Child Abuse & Neglect*, *17*(6), 843–854.

Almqvist, K., & Brandell-Forsberg, M. (1997). Refugee children in Sweden: Posttraumatic stress disorder in Iranian preschool children exposed to organized violence. *Child Abuse & Neglect*, *21*(4), 351–366.

Almqvist, K., & Broberg, A. G. (1999). Mental health and social adjustment in young refugee children 3½ years after their arrival in Sweden. *Journal of the American Academy of Child & Adolescent Psychiatry, 38*(6), 723.

Baarnhielm, S., & Mosko, M. (2015). Cross-cultural communication with traumatised immigrants. In M. Schouler-Ocak (Ed.), *Trauma and migration* (pp. 39–56). Basel, Switzerland: Springer International.

Birman, D., & Chan, W. Y. (2008). Screening and assessing immigrant and refugee youth in school-based mental health programs. Center for Health and Health Care in Schools. Issue Brief 1. https://www.rwjf.org/en/library/research/2008/05/screening-and-assessing-immigrant-and-refugee-youth-in-school-ba.html.

Bodegard, G. (2005). Life-threatening loss of function in refugee children: Another expression of pervasive refusal syndrome? *Clinical Child Psychology and Psychiatry, 10*(3), 337–350.

Bogic, M., Njoku, A., & Priebe, S. (2015). Long-term mental health of war-refugees: A systematic literature review. *International Health and Human Rights, 15*, article 29.) https://bmcinthealthhumrights.biomedcentral.com/articles/10.1186/s12914-015-0064-9. Accessed June 6, 2018.

Bolton, P., Lee, C., Haroz, E. E., et al. (2014). A transdiagnostic community-based mental health treatment for comorbid disorders: Development and outcomes of a randomized controlled trial among Burmese refugees in Thailand. *PloS Medicine, 11*(11). 1–16. http://journals.plos.org/plosmedicine/article?id=10.1371/journal.pmed.1001757. Accessed June 14, 2018.

Boothby, N. (1994). Trauma and violence among refugee children. In A. Marsella, S. Bornemann, J. Ekblad, & J. Orley (Eds.), *Amidst peril and pain: The mental health and well-being of the world's refugees*. Washington, DC: American Psychological Association.

Brofenbrenner, U. (1979). *The ecology of human development: Experiments by nature and design*. Cambridge, MA: Harvard University Press.

Cohen, J., and the Work Group on Quality Issues of the American Academy of Child and Adolescent Psychiatry. (2010). Practice parameter for the assessment and treatment of children and adolescents with posttraumatic stress disorder. *Journal of the American Academy of Child and Adolescent Psychiatry, 49*(4), 414–430. https://www.jaacap.org/article/S0890-8567(10)00082-1/pdf. Accessed June 14, 2018.

Chimienti, G., Nasr, J. A., & Khalifeh, I. (1989). Children's reactions to war-related stress. *Social Psychiatry and Psychiatric Epidemiology, 24*, 282–287.

Chow, J., Jaffee, K., & Choi, D. (1999). Use of public mental health services by Russian refugees. *Psychiatric Services, 50*(7), 936–940.

Curry, J., Rohe, P., Simons, A., et al. (2006). Predictors and modifiers of acute outcome in the Treatment for Adolescents with Depression Study (TADS). *Journal of the American Academy of Child and Adolescent Psychiatry, 45*, 1427–1439.

De Antiss, H., Ziaian, T., Procter, N., Warland, J., & Baghurst, P. (2009). Help-seeking for mental health problems in young refugees: A review of the literature with implications for policy, practice, and research. *Transcultural Psychiatry, 46*(4), 584–607.

Dossa, P. (2002). Narrative mediation of conventional and new "mental health" paradigms: Reading the stories of immigrant Iranian women. *Medical Anthropology Quarterly, 16*(3), 341–359.

Dyregrov, A., Gupta, L., Gjestad, R., & Mukanoheli, E. (2000). Trauma exposure and psychological reactions to genocide among Rwandan children. *Journal of Traumatic Stress, 13*, 3–21.

Ehntholt, K. A. (2005). School-based cognitive-behavioural therapy group intervention for refugee children who have experienced war-related trauma. *Clinical Child Psychology and Psychiatry, 10*(2), 235–250.

Ehntholt, K. A., & Yule, W. (2006). Practitioner review: Assessment and treatment of refugee children and adolescents who have experienced war related trauma. *Journal of Child Psychology and Psychiatry, 47*(12), 1197–1210.

Ehntholt, K. A., Smith, P. A., & Yule, W. (2005). School-based Cognitive-Behavioural Therapy Group Intervention for Refugee Children who have Experienced War-related Trauma *Clinical Child Psychology and Psychiatry, 10*(2), 235–250.

Fahy, T. A., Robinson, P. H., Russell, G. F., & Sheinman, B. (1988). Anorexia nervosa following torture in a young African woman. *British Journal of Psychiatry, 153*, 385–387.

Fazel, M., Wheeler, J., & Danesh, J. (2005). Prevalence of serious mental disorder in 7000 refugees resettled in Western countries: A systematic review. *Lancet, 365*(9467), 1309–1314.

Felsman, J. K., Leong, F. T. L., Johnson, M. C., & Felsman, I. C. (1990). Estimates of psychological distress among Vietnamese refugees: Adolescents, unaccompanied minors and young adults. *Social Science and Medicine, 31*, 1251–1256.

Fox, P. G., Cowell, J. M., & Montgomery, A. C. (1994). The effects of violence on health and adjustment of Southeast Asian refugee children: An integrative review. *Public Health Nursing, 11*, 195–201.

Garmezy, N., & Rutter, M. (1985). Acute reactions to stress. In M. Rutter & L. Hersov (Eds.), *Child and adolescent psychiatry, modern approaches* (2nd ed., pp. 152–176). Oxford, England: Blackwell.

Heaphy, G., Ehntholt, K., & Sclare, I. (2007). Groupwork with unaccompanied young women. In R. Kohli & F. Mitchell (Eds.), *Social work with unaccompanied asylum seeking children: Practice and policy issues* (pp. 77–94). Basingstoke, England: Palgrave.

Hjern, A., & Angel, B. (2000). Organized violence and mental health of refugee children in exile: A six-year follow-up. *Acta Paediatrica, 89*(6), 722–727.

Hjern, A., Angel, B., & Hojer, B. (1991). Persecution and behavior: A report of refugee children from Chile. *Child Abuse & Neglect, 15*(3), 239–248.

Hodes, M. (1998). Refugee children may need a lot of psychiatric help. *British Medical Journal, 316*(7134), 793–794.

Hodes M. (2000). Psychologically distressed refugee children in the United Kingdom. *Child Psychology & Psychiatry Review, 5*(2), 57–68.

Hodes, M. (2002). Three key issues for young refugees' mental health. *Transcultural Psychiatry, 39*(2), 196–213.

Hodes, M., & Tolmac, J. (2005). Severely impaired young refugees. *Clinical Child Psychology and Psychiatry, 10*(2), 251–261.

Hollifield, M., Warner, T. D., Lian, N., et al. (2002). Measuring trauma and health status in refugees: A critical review. *Journal of the American Medical Association, 288*(5), 611–621.

Howard, M., & Hodes, M. (2000). Psychopathology, adversity, and service utilization of young refugees. *Journal of the American Academy of Child and Adolescent Psychiatry, 39*(3), 368–377.

Human Rights Watch. (2018). Child soldiers. https://www.hrw.org/topic/childrens-rights/child-soldiers. Accessed June 9, 2018.

Kataoka, S., Stein, B., Jaycox, L., et al. (2003). A school-based mental health program for traumatized Latino immigrant children. *Journal of the American Academy of Child and Adolescent Psychiatry, 42*, 311–318.

Keely, C. B. (1996). How nation-states create and respond to refugee flows. *International Migration Review, 30*, 1046–1066.

Kinzie, J. D. (2006). Immigrants and refugees: The psychiatric perspective. *Transcultural Psychiatry, 43*(4), 577–591.

Kinzie, J. D., & Leung, P. (1989). Clonidine in Cambodian patients with posttraumatic stress disorder. *Journal of Nervous and Mental Disease, 177*, 546–550.

Kinzie, J. D., Sack, W. H., Angell, R., & Clarke, G. N. (1989). A three-year follow-up of Cambodian young people traumatized as children. *Journal of the American Academy of Child & Adolescent Psychiatry, 28*(4), 501–504.

Kinzie, J. D., Sack, W. H., Angell, R. H., Manson, S., & Rath, B. (1986). The psychiatric effects of massive trauma on Cambodian children: 1. The children. *Journal of the American Academy of Child and Adolescent Psychiatry, 25*(3), 370–376.

Kirmayer, L., Groleau, D., Guzder, J., Blake, C., & Jarvis, E. (2003). Cultural consultation: A model of mental health service for multicultural societies. *Canadian Journal of Psychiatry, 48*(3),145–153.

Kleinman, A. (1987). Anthropology and psychiatry: The role of culture in crosscultural research on illness. *British Journal of Psychiatry, 151*, 447–454.

Krupinski, J., & Burrows, G. D. (1986). *The price of freedom: Young Indochinese refugees in Australia*. Sydney, Australia: Pergamon Press.

Kuey, L. (2015). Trauma and migration: The role of stigma. In M. Schouler-Ocak (Ed.), *Trauma and migration* (pp. 57–68). Basel, Switzerland: Springer International.

Laban, C. J., Gernaat, H. P. B. E., Komproe, I. H., & De Jong, J. T. V. M. (2007). Prevalence and predictors of health service use among Iraqi asylum seekers in the Netherlands. *Social Psychiatry and Psychiatric Epidemiology, 42*, 837–844.

Laban, C. J., Gernaat, H. B. P. E., Komproe, I. H., Schreuders, G. A., & De Jong, J. T. V. M. (2004). Impact of a long asylum procedure on the prevalence of psychiatric disorders in Iraqi asylum seekers in the Netherlands. *The Journal of Nervous and Mental Disease,192*(12), 843–885.

Laban, C. J., Gernaat, H. B. P. E., Komproe, I. H., Van Tweel, I., & De Jong, J. T. V. M. (2005). Post migration living problems and common psychiatric disorders in Iraqi asylum seekers in the Netherlands. *The Journal of Nervous and Mental Disease, 193*(12), 825–832.

Layne, C. M., Pynoos, R. S., Saltzman, W. R., et al. (2001). Trauma/grief-focused group psychotherapy: School-based postwar intervention with traumatized Bosnian adolescents. *Group Dynamics: Theory, Research and Practice*, *5*, 277–290.

Lindert, J., Ehrenstein, O. S., Priebe, S., Mielck, A., & Brahler, E. (2009). Depression and anxiety in labor migrants and refugees: A systematic review and meta-analysis. *Social Science and Medicine*, *69*(2), 246–257.

Lurie, I., & Nakash, O. (2015). Exposure to trauma and forced migration: Mental health and acculturation patterns among asylum seekers in Israel. In M. Schouler-Ocak (Ed.), *Trauma and migration* (pp. 139–158). Basel, Switzerland: Springer International.

Lustig, S. L., Kia-Keating, M., Knight, W. G., et al. (2004). Review of child and adolescent refugee mental health. *Journal of the American Academy of Child and Adolescent Psychiatry*, *43*(1), 24–36.

Lustig, S. L., Weine, S. M., Saxe, G. N., & Beardslee, W. R. (2004). Testimonial psychotherapy for adolescent refugees: A case series. *Transcultural Psychiatry*, *41*, 31–45.

McKelvey, R. S., Sang, D. L., Baldassar, L., Davies, L., Roberts, L., & Cutler, N. (2002). The prevalence of psychiatric disorders among Vietnamese children and adolescents. *Medical Journal of Australia*, *177*(8), 413–417.

McKelvey, R. S., & Webb, J. A. (1995). Unaccompanied status as a risk factor in Vietnamese Amerasians. *Social Science and Medicine*, *41*, 261–266.

Mghir, R., Freed, W., Raskin, A., & Katon, W. (1995). Depression and posttraumatic stress disorder among a community sample of adolescent and young adult Afghan refugees. *Journal of Nervous and Mental Disease*, *183*, 24–30.

Minas, H., & Sawyer, S. M. (2002). The mental health of immigrant and refugee children and adolescents. *The Medical Journal of Australia*, *177*(8), 404–405.

Mollica, R. F., Cui, X., McInnes, K., & Massagli, M. (2002). Science-based policy for psychosocial interventions in refugee camps: A Cambodian example. *Journal of Nervous and Mental Disease*, *190*(3), 158–166.

Mollica, R. F., Poole, C., Son, L., & Murray, C. C. (1997). Effects of war trauma on Cambodian refugee adolescents' functional health and mental health status. *Journal of the American Academy of Child & Adolescent Psychiatry*, *36*(8), 1098–1106.

Nader, K., Pynoos, R. S., Fairbanks, L., Al-Ajeel, M., & Al-Asfour, A. (1993). A preliminary study of PTSD and grief among the children of Kuwait following the Gulf crisis. *British Journal of Clinical Psychology*, *32*, 407–416.

The National Center for Mental Health Promotion and Youth Violence Prevention at Education Development Center. (2011). Strategies for engaging immigrant and refugee families. http://www.redincola.org/en/download_fic.php?id=6. Accessed June 12, 2018.

Nicholli, C., & Thompson, A. (2004). The psychological treatment of post-traumatic stress disorder (PTSD) in adult refugees: A review of the current state of psychological therapies *Journal of Mental Health*, *13*(4): 351–362.

Nurussaman, M. (2009). Revisiting the category of fragile and failed states in international relations. *International Studies*, *46*(3), 271–294.

Onyut, L. P., Neuner, F., Schauer, E., et al. (2005). Narrative exposure therapy as a treatment for child war survivors with posttraumatic stress disorder: Two case reports and a pilot study in an African settlement. *BMC Psychiatry*, *5*, 1–9.

Oras, R., Cancela de Ezpeleta, S., &Ahmad, A. (2004). Treatment of traumatized refugee children with eye movement desensitization and reprocessing in a psychodynamic context. *Nordic Journal of Psychiatry, 58*, 199–203.

Ozkan, I., & Belz, M. (2015). Clinical diagnosis of traumatized children. In M. Schouler-Ocak (Ed.), *Trauma and migration* (pp. 83–94). Basel, Switzerland: Springer International.

Papageorgiou, V., Frangou-Garunovic, A., Iordanidou, R., Yule, W., Smith, P., & Vostanis, P. (2000). War trauma and psychopathology in Bosnian refugee children. *European Child and Adolescent Psychiatry, 9*, 84–90.

Patel, N., & Hodes, M. (2006). Violent deliberate self-harm amongst adolescent refugees. *European Child & Adolescent Psychiatry, 15*(6), 367–370.

Pedersen, D. (2015). Rethinking trauma as a global challenge. In M. Schouler-Ocak (Ed.), *Trauma and migration* (pp. 9–32). Basel, Switzerland: Springer International.

Phan, T. (2000). Investigating the use of services for Vietnamese with mental illness. *Journal of Community Health, 25*(5), 411–425.

Porter, M., & Haslam, N. (2005). Predisplacement and postdisplacement factors associated with mental health of refugees and internally displaced persons: A meta-analysis. *JAMA, 294*(5), 602–612.

Pumariega, A. J., Glover, S., Holzer, C. E., & Nguyen, N. (1998). Utilization of mental health services in a tri-ethnic sample of adolescents. *Community Mental Health Journal, 34*(2), 145–156.

Pumariega, A., Rogers, K., & Rothe, E. (2005). Culturally competent systems of care for children's mental health: Advances and challenges. *Community Mental Health Journal, 41*, 539–556.

Pumariega, A., Rothe, E. M., Mian, A., et al. (2013). Practice parameters for cultural competence in child psychiatric practice. *Journal of the American Academy of Child and Adolescent Psychiatry, 52*(12), 1101–1115.

Pumariega, A. J., Rothe, E. M., & Pumariega, J. A. (2005). Mental health issues in immigrant and refugee children in the United States. *Community Mental Health Journal, 41*(5), 581–597.

Pumariega, A. J., Rothe, E., & Rogers, K. (2009). Cultural competence in child psychiatric practice. *Journal of the American Academy of Child and Adolescent Psychiatry, 48*(4), 362–366.

Punamäki, R. L. (1996). Can ideological commitment protect children's psychosocial well-being in situations of political violence? *Child Development, 67*, 55–69.

Rechtman, R. (2000). Stories of trauma and idioms of distress: From cultural narratives to clinical assessment. *Transcultural Psychiatry, 37*(3), 403–415.

Rose, P. I. (2014). Refugees defined. In F. Bean & S. Brown. (Eds.), *Encyclopedia of migration*. Dordrecht, Netherlands: Springer.

Rothbaum, B. O., Foa, E. B., Riggs, D. S., Murdock, T., & Walsh, W. (1992). A prospective examination of post-traumatic stress disorder in rape victims. *Journal of Traumatic Stress, 5*, 455–475.

Rothe, E. M. (2005). Post-traumatic stress symptoms in Cuban children and adolescents during and after refugee camp confinement. In T.A. Corales (Ed.), *Trends in post-traumatic stress disorder research*. New York: Nova Science.

Rothe, E. M. (2008). A psychotherapy model for treating refugee children caught in the midst of catastrophic situations. *Journal of the American Academy of Psychoanalysis and Dynamic Psychiatry, 36*, 625–642.

Rothe, E. M., Castillo, H., Lewis, J., Martinez, O., Gonzalez, C. M., Busquets, R., . . . Aranguren, E. (1998). Sintomatologia Post-Traumatica en Ninos y Adolecentes Balseros Cubanos: Una Sinopsis de Tres Estudios. (Post-Traumatic Symptomatology in Child and Adolescent Cuban Boat Children: A Synopsis of Three Studies) *Psiquiatria*. Madrid, Spain. (Jan-Feb).

Rothe, E. M., Castillo-Matos, H., Brinson, K., & Lewis, J. (2000). La Odisea de los Balseros Cubanos: Sintomas Post-traumaticos y Caracteristicas de Viaje en Niños y Adolescentes (The Odissey of the Cuban Rafters: Post-Traumatic Symptomatology in Children and Adolescents). *Medico Interamericano, 19*(12).

Rothe, E. M., Castillo-Matos, H., & Busquets R. (2002). Post-traumatic stress symptoms in Cuban adolescent refugees during camp confinement. *Adolescent Psychiatry, 26*, 97–124.

Rothe, E. M., Lewis, J., Castillo-Matos, H., Martinez, O., Busquets, R., & Martinez, I. (2002). Posttraumatic stress disorder among Cuban children and adolescents after release from a refugee camp. *Psychiatric Services, 53*(8), 970–976.

Rothe, E. M., & Pumariega, A. J. (2012). Mental health issues of child and adolescent refugees. In U. Segal, D. Elliott, & N. Mayadas (Eds.), *Immigration worldwide: Policies, practices, and trends* (Chapter 5, pp. 81–108). New York: Oxford University Press.

Rothe, E. M., Tzuang, D., & Pumariega, A. J. (2010). Acculturation, development and adaptation. *Child and Adolescent Psychiatry Clinics of North America, 19*(4), 681–696.

Rousseau, C. (1995). The mental health of refugee children. *Transcultural Psychiatric Research Review, 32*(3), 299–331.

Rousseau, C., & Drapeau, A. (2003). Are refugee children an at-risk group? A longitudinal study of Cambodian adolescents. *Journal of Refugee Studies, 16*(1), 67–81.

Rousseau, C., Drapeau, A., & Corin, E. (1996). School performance and emotional problems in refugee children. *American Journal of Orthopsychiatry, 66*(2), 239–251.

Rousseau, C., & Guzder, J. (2008). School-based prevention programs for refugee children. *Child and Adolescent Clinics of North America, 17*, 533–549.

Sack, W. H., Clarke, G. N., Him, C., Dickason, D., Goff, B., Lanham, K., & Kinzie, J. D. (1993). A 6-year follow-up study of Cambodian refugee adolescents traumatized as children. *Journal of the American Academy of Child and Adolescent Psychiatry, 32*, 431–437.

Sack, W. H., Clarke, G. N., & Seeley, J. (1996). Multiple forms of stress in Cambodian adolescent refugees. *Child Development, 67*(1), 107–116.

Sack, W. H., Him, C., & Dickason, D. (1999). Twelve-year follow-up study of Khmer youths who suffered massive war trauma as children. *Journal of the American Academy of Child & Adolescent Psychiatry, 38*(9), 1173.

Sack, W. H., McSharry, S., Clarke, G. N., Kinney, R., Seeley, J., & Lewinsohn, P. (1994). The Khmer adolescent project. I. Epidemiological findings in two generations of Cambodian refugees. *Journal of Nervous and Mental Disease, 182*, 387–395.

Sack, W. H., Seeley, J. R., & Clarke, G. N. (1997). Does PTSD transcend cultural barriers? A study from the Khmer adolescent refugee project. *Journal of the American Academy of Child and Adolescent Psychiatry, 36*, 49–54.

Schnauer, E., & Elbert, E. (2010). The psychological impact of child soldering. In A. H. Eide (Ed.), *Trauma rehabilitation after war and conflict: Community and individual perspectives* (pp. 311–360). New York: Springer. https://www.researchgate.net/publication/230651547_The_Psychological_Impact_of_Child_Soldiering. Accessed June 9, 2018.

Seligman, M. E., & Csikszentmihalyi, M. (2000). Positive psychology: An introduction. *American Psychologist, 55*(1), 5–14.

Servan-Schreiber, D., Le Lin, B., & Birmaher, B. (1998). Prevalence of posttraumatic stress disorder and major depressive disorder in Tibetan refugee children. *Journal of the American Academy of Child and Adolescent Psychiatry, 37*(8), 874–879.

Shannon, P. J., Im, H., Becher, E., Simmelink, J., Wieling, E., & O'Fallon, A. (2012). Screening for war trauma, torture, and mental health symptoms among newly arrived refugees: A national survey of U.S. refugee health coordinators. *Journal of Immigrant & Refugee Studies, 10*, 380–394.

Shannon, P. J., Weiling, E., Simmelink-McCleary, E., & Becher, E. (2015). Exploring the effects of political trauma with newly arrived refugees. *Qualitative Health Research, 25*(4), 443–457.

Shoeb, M., Weinstein, H., & Mollica, R. (2007). The Harvard Trauma Questionnaire: Adapting a cross-cultural instrument for measuring torture, trauma and posttraumatic stress disorder in Iraqi refugees. *International Journal of Social Psychiatry, 53*(5), 447–463.

Silove, D. (1999). The psychosocial effects of torture, mass human rights violations, and refugee trauma: Toward an integrated conceptual framework. *Journal of Nervous and Mental Disease, 187*(4), 200–207.

Silove, D. (2005). From trauma to survival and adaptation. In D. Ingleby (Ed.), *Forced migration and mental health: Rethinking the care of refugees and displaced persons* (pp. 29–51). Utrecht, Netherlands: Springer.

Simich, L., Beiser, M., & Mawani, F. (2003). Social support and the significance of shared experience in refugee migration and resettlement. *Western Journal of Nursing Research, 25*(7), 872–891.

Small, E., Kim, Y. K., Praetorius, R. T., & Mitschke, D. B. (2016). Mental health treatment for resettled refugees: A comparison of three approaches. *Social Work in Mental Health, 14*(4), 342–359.

Smith, P., Perrin, S., Yule, W., Hacam, B., & Stuvland, R. (2002). War exposure among children from Bosnia-Hercegovina: Psychological adjustment in a community sample. *Journal of Traumatic Stress, 15*, 147–156.

Sourander, A. (1998). Behavior problems and traumatic events of unaccompanied refugee minors. *Child Abuse & Neglect, 22*(7), 719–727.

Summerfield, D. (1995). Addressing human response to war and atrocity: Major challenges in research and practices and the limitations of Western psychiatric models. In R. J. Kleber, C. R. Figley, & B. P. R. Gersons (Eds.), *Beyond trauma: Cultural and societal dynamics* (pp. 17–29). New York: Plenum Press.

Summerfield, D. (1999). A critique of seven assumptions behind psychological trauma programmes in war-affected areas. *Social Science and Medicine, 48*, 1449–1462.

Summerfield, D. (2000). Childhood, war, refugeedom and "trauma": Three core questions for mental health professionals. *Transcultural Psychiatry, 37*(3), 417.

Summerfield, D. (2003). Mental health of refugees. *The British Journal of Psychiatry, 183*, 459–460.

Steel, Z., Silove, D., Phan, T., & Bauman, A. (2002). Long-term effect of psychological trauma on the mental health of Vietnamese refugees resettled in Australia: A population based study. *Lancet, 360*, 1056–1062.

Thabet, A. A. M., & Vostanis, P. (1999). Post-traumatic stress reactions in children of war. *Journal of Child Psychology and Psychiatry, 40*, 385–391.

Thomas, S., Thomas, S., Nafees, B., & Bhugra, D. (2004). "I was running away from death"—The preflight experiences of unaccompanied asylum seeking children in the UK. *Child: Care, Health and Development, 30*, 113–122.

Tolmac, J., & Hodes, M. (2004). Ethnic variation among adolescent psychiatric inpatients with psychotic disorders. *British Journal of Psychiatry, 184*, 428–431.

Tousignant, M., Habimana, E., Biron, C., Malo, C., Sidoli-LeBlanc, E., & Bendris, N. (1999). The Quebec adolescent refugee project: Psychopathology and family variables in a sample from 35 nations. *Journal of the American Academy of Child & Adolescent Psychiatry, 38*(11), 1426–1432.

Tseng, W. (2001). *Handbook of cultural psychiatry*. San Diego, CA: Academic Press.

United Nations High Commissioner for Refugees (UNHCR). (2016). Global trends: Forced displacement in 2016. https://www.unhcr.org/5943e8a34.pdf. Accessed June 4, 2018.

Von Folsach, L. L., & Montgomery, E. (2006). Pervasive refusal syndrome among asylum-seeking children. *Clinical Child Psychology and Psychiatry, 11*(3), 457–473.

Watters, C. (2001). Emerging paradigms in the mental health care of refugees. *Social Science & Medicine, 52*(11), 1709.

Weine, S. M., Kulenovic, T., Dzubur, A., Pavkovic, I., & Gibbons, R. (1998). Testimony psychotherapy in Bosnian refugees: A pilot study. *American Journal of Psychiatry, 155*, 1720–1726.

Westermeyer, J., & Janca, A. (1997). Language, culture and psychopathology: Conceptual and methodological issues. *Transcultural Psychiatry, 34*, 291–311.

Williams, C. L., & Westermeyer, J. (1983). Psychiatric problems among adolescent Southeast Asian refugees: A descriptive study. *Journal of Nervous and Mental Disease, 171*(2), 79–85.

Zarowsky, C. (2000). Trauma stories: Violence, emotion and politics in Somali Ethiopia. *Transcultural Psychiatry, 37*(3), 383–402.

7

Transnational Identities, Pilgrimages, and Return Migrations

The concept of *transnationalism* refers to multiple interactions that link people and institutions across national borders. In the twenty-first century, the development of new communication technologies and the easy and affordable access to international transportation has dramatically changed the relationship between people and places. It is now possible for immigrants to maintain closer and more frequent contact with their home societies than ever before. Transnationalism is part of a process of capitalist globalization in which citizens of many developing countries fill not only the demand for low-wage workers in more developed countries, but also, at times, the demographic gaps created by declining natural populations in the more industrialized countries.

Transnational migration refers to the process by which many immigrants now live their lives in more than one country and have to negotiate alternating national and cultural norms. In addition to the country to which they have immigrated, many remain active in their countries of origin, transforming the politics, the economy, cultural norms such as gender relations, and other aspects of everyday life. They send remittances back home and create three distinct categories of experience: (1) those who migrate, (2) those who stay behind and receive financial support from the relatives who migrated, and (3) those who do not migrate and have no sources of outside support. Sometimes, monetary remittances to the home country are seen as a double-edged sword; on the one hand, they improve the economic conditions of those who receive them, but they are also seen as responsible for creating materialistic and individualistic attitudes that erode the traditional values of extended family and community. Remittances are not only monetary, but also include *social remittances*, which involve the exchange of ideas about democracy, gender equality, health, and community organization that deeply impact the immigrant's country of origin.

A curious case of transnationalism has been that of Puerto Rico; because Puerto Ricans are considered American citizens, they move freely back and forth between the island and the mainland without the migratory restrictions faced by migrants of other nationalities. This type of *shuttle migration* does not cross political borders, but the Puerto Rican migrants cross significant cultural, linguistic, and geographic borders and differ from other immigrants to the U.S. mainland due to the island's nebulous definition as an unincorporated territory (Duany, 2011).

Transnational attitudes are most important for the first generation of immigrants and tend to fade in subsequent generations; however, many of the children that are being raised in transnational households are raised in homes saturated by influences from the countries of origin of their parents or grandparents. These children may choose to activate and identify with their ancestral cultural identities at any given time if they find that this can be useful to them. In addition, many economists argue that rather than seeing remittances as a drain to the U.S. economy, they should be seen as a way to spread the wealth of nations in a way that rectifies years of uneven economic development and guarantees global political stability (Levitt, 2001, 2004).

Children of transnational immigrants also contribute to the process of *interculturation* in the schools they attend. Students who are native born and those who are the children of immigrants exchange ideas in which both groups acquire a better understanding and greater appreciation of diverse languages, customs, and beliefs. This contributes to creating an openness and fluidity that are necessary to develop citizens of a global society. In turn, for children of immigrant families who are struggling to move out of poverty and into the middle class, a sense of school belonging serves as a buffer against the lack of *neighborhood space*. In current times, when xenophobic and anti-immigrant rhetoric is increasing in news headlines and in political speeches, public schools in the United States serve the vital function of providing a space where the future generations of students can learn to trust one another and experience what it means to be part of a community working in pursuit of common goals (Keegan, 2017).

RETURN MIGRATIONS

Return migration is defined as the movement of immigrants back to their homelands to resettle. In the last 200 years, massive industrialization took place in the United States, so most immigrants arriving during this period came from rural areas and moved into industrialized centers where they obtained unskilled jobs that, nevertheless, paid more than what they were making at home. They followed a chain of immigration, usually settling in places where their kinsmen had already become established. Return migration is probably the aspect of the migration cycle that has been granted the lowest attention, perhaps because most research resources are located in highly developed countries, while most returnees return to developing countries. In the early part of the twentieth century, it is estimated that approximately 4 million Europeans returned to their home countries after immigrating to the United States, yet these were barely noticed by social scientists.

Among people who return to their countries of origin, there are those who intended their migration to be temporary, searching to accomplish a particular objective, usually financial improvement, and there were those who intended it to be permanent. The latter mostly sought to create a better life abroad for themselves and for their families. Various reasons are given for returning: (1) The person achieved the objective set for him- or herself; (2) the person wished to stay but was forced to return due to external factors; (3) new opportunities appeared in the person's home country that were favorable to the skills and experiences acquired abroad; and (4) there are those who intended to stay but were unable to adjust due to cultural issues or homesickness. Occasionally, return migrations occur when there are negative push factors, which include, among others, an unexpected encounter of the immigrant with racial discrimination, economic recessions that make employment difficult in the host country, or, like the case of many Puerto Ricans in the 1960s, displacement from factory jobs by automation and mechanization caused a return to the island. Research findings have shown that most immigrants do not have any definitive plans for the future but decide their fate given the available opportunities (Gmelch, 1980).

In terms of education, return migration follows a U-shaped curve, with those returning being in both extremes of the education spectrum, the most and the least well educated. Return migration is greater between countries with similar levels of development, but when income disparities are greater, people tend to stay in the host country (Dumont & Spielvogel, 2008).

Interestingly, empirical studies showed that the reintegration in the country of origin is not exactly a smooth one (Pirvu & Axinte, 2012). Many migrants are ill prepared for their return and are not always aware of the rapid changes that took place in their former homelands, even when there has been intense communication with other family members in their community of origin. They often do not realize how much their communities changed during their absence. Also, the migrant who returned home after 10 or 20 years of residence in another country is not the same as the person who left the country because the immigrant is now in a different life stage and, perhaps without personal awareness, the values, goals, and expectations of the immigrant have been transformed by a life experience different from the one of those that were left behind. Those returning from industrialized nations to rural developing countries no longer share many of the basic notions that underlie their traditional cultures, their relatives and former friends no longer share the same interests, and the returning migrant may find that former close friends seem narrow, provincial, and backward. Local people have developed new friendships during the years that the migrant was absent and are not always enthusiastic about resuming old relationships. Returning migrants often experience a form of *reverse culture shock* and discover, to their surprise, that now they have more in common with the people of the host society than with the people in their former country.

Case I

A Latin American physician who came to the United States in his mid-20s to complete postgraduate work had initial plans of returning to his home country to practice medicine after completing his medical specialty training. However, he married an American woman and found attractive professional opportunities in the host country, where he formed a family and has been practicing medicine for over 30y years. During a visit to his country of origin, where he harbored fantasies of someday retiring, he was horrified when one of his sisters commented in a conversation that, "We have to be careful with our youth in this country because there is a bar downtown where they put a drug in the drinks, and the children turn into homosexuals." Incredulous, the physician attempted to explain to his sister, a university graduate, that this was not scientifically possible, that it was almost certain that homosexually had a biological origin. He asked her if she had considered that the place was possibly a gay bar, but she persevered in her argument, stating that, "People around town are saying it's true because more than one young man or woman has come out of there being gay, when in actuality they were not gay before." Astounded, he commented to a colleague on returning to the United States, "I could never go back to live in a place like that where people are so backward and close-minded."

In some cases, returning migrants encounter envy and suspicion among their less prosperous neighbors and find that locals try to take advantage of them by overcharging higher wages for services. The most frequent complaints center on issues of inefficiency and lack of punctuality because the returning migrant has become accustomed at life in in urban industrial societies where the pace of life is much faster. For many returning migrants, memories of the home country where they were socialized are often nostalgic and idealized; the negative memories are forgotten and recede into the background. The times lived in the home country often took place during the migrant's younger years, when life was more carefree and devoid of adult responsibilities. Vacation visits are not representative of the realities of the home country because they are undertaken in a celebratory and festive atmosphere, with the joys of reencounter with only the positives highlighted. The farewells often leave the migrant with a feeling of emotional deprivation and longing for the emotional closeness and joy that were experienced during those brief reencounters.

For most, their reasons to return are centered on strong family ties, responsibility to care for elderly relatives, and the desire to be among one's kin and longtime friends. The dream of most returning immigrants who worked as unskilled laborers in the host country is to return to their home countries and be self-employed and financially independent, opening up small businesses such as a grocery store, or to retire and live off their savings and the retirement benefits they acquired during the long years of work and sacrifice away from home. Yet, for the most part, returning migrants who have been financially successful are usually seen in a very positive light by their compatriots and are held as role models (Gmelch, 1980).

PILGRIMAGES

A pilgrimage, in its more traditional form, is a journey to a distant place that is sacred and venerable for some reason, undertaken for devotional purposes (Poland, 1977). The history of pilgrimages antedates the genesis of the four major world religions, and these journeys have played a crucial role throughout human history, enhancing cultural contact and disseminating goods and novel ideas. Human beings are faced in their lives with the duality of *liminality* (or in-betweenness). They alternate geographically between that which is close and familiar, defined by the German word *Heimweh* and that which is distant, inaccessible and longed for, known as *Fernweh*.

Throughout our human history, pilgrimages to symbolic places become the basis for the regeneration of personal values and the reconstruction of personal and cultural identities (Beckstead, 2010). They provide a time away from the mundane and are valuable in creating deep bonds between the self and others and with the site of the pilgrimage. They produce narratives that explore human motivations, fears, hopes, and dreams and help to illuminate the human soul. Many times, they serve to break down barriers between classes, religions, ethnicities, and genders and to highlight what is authentic in our human experience (Warfield, Baker, & Parikh-Foxx, 2014).

In the case of immigrants or their descendants, pilgrimages are particularly valuable in mastering conscious and unconscious identifications with members of the previous generations. The immigrant, or descendant of an immigrant, struggles to integrate previously unmastered identifications in order to establish his or her personal identity as an individual, simultaneously attempting to master and integrate a cultural identity that has been passed down by the previous generations of this family and to make the continuity from one generation to another more conflict free (Poland, 1977). The importance of pilgrimages is evidenced by the pervasiveness of the phenomenon in all cultures throughout history.

In addition to actual travels, a pilgrimage refers to any major journey in life, including the actual person's life journey from birth to death. Psychoanalysis, psychotherapy, and other journeys of self-reflection, self-exploration, and self-discovery are also defined as pilgrimages. Certain characteristics, either actual or symbolic, are common to all pilgrimages. The pilgrimage is a journey that is difficult, demanding work and sacrifice, usually covering long distances. The pilgrim goes in search of spiritual or personal change. The assimilation and identification of these new introjects leads to new levels of self-integration with a shift of one's sense of self.

Case II

Seth, a successful and very assertive trial lawyer considered himself to be a warrior who always went into the courtroom "to win and take no prisoners." Seth's father was a child survivor of the Holocaust and suffered symptoms of severe post-traumatic stress disorder, which made him moody, irritable, aloof, and unable to express affection to his son. Seth was unable to connect emotionally with his father, who never complimented his son's successes and always told him that, "nothing in your life will ever compare to what I had to go through." Seth was also very ambivalent about his Jewish identity and despised the image of Jews as victims. His childhood hero was Moshe Dayan (a fighting Jew), the gallant Israeli general with an eyepatch who helped reconquer Jerusalem during the Six Day War of 1967. After the death of his father, Seth felt very conflicted with the fact that they had never been able to achieve any kind of emotional closeness. After a year of work in psychotherapy, he embarked on a pilgrimage to the sites of the concentration camps of Auschwitz and Buchenwald, where his father had been interned and where most of Seth's extended family was murdered. The experience was a very powerful one, and on his return, Seth reported that he felt "transformed." In the course of the following year in therapy, he mourned the losses of the many relatives he had never met, and he also began to reconceptualize the image of his father. This time, he no longer saw his father as a victim, but as "a survivor" and spoke about him as a man of great resiliency, determination, and inner strength. Seth also began to develop a newfound pride in his Jewish identity.

Case III

Anthony, a very successful business executive, arrived from Cuba at the age of 11 as an unaccompanied refugee child. In 1961, at the height of the Cold War and after Cuba had become a communist country, his parents were forbidden to leave because they were both physicians, but they feared that if Anthony stayed in Cuba, he would be forcefully sent to a communist boarding school and later conscripted into the military. So, Anthony was sent to the United States to be cared for by maternal relatives who had established themselves in New York City prior to the Communist Revolution in Cuba. As a result of his efforts, talent, and ambition, Anthony obtained merit scholarships in high school, graduated from a prestigious university, and became very successful professionally and financially. He integrated wholeheartedly into the northeastern U.S. establishment, married an Anglo-American wife, and even Americanized his first name. Anthony reunited with his parents more than 10 years later when he was already in his 20s; by that time, he had already left the home of his relatives and was living independently. A few years after his parents arrived in the United States, a role reversal occurred in which he began to provide financially for his parents, and for most of the remaining years of their lives, it was Anthony who played the parental role vis-à-vis his parents. Anthony was living in Miami when his marriage began to fail, and he was feeling desolate and confused and had fallen into a deep state of depression. He sought psychiatric help and, in the course of psychotherapy, began to explore his many unmourned losses. He rediscovered that the only parental figure he had ever deeply loved was his Cuban nanny, who had stayed behind on the island, and he had never seen her again. Anthony had always silently longed for her, but never spoke about this and had kept these feelings as a well-kept secret. After months of planning, Anthony embarked on a pilgrimage to the island of Cuba to find his nanny. Once in Cuba, he visited the sites of his childhood and contacted the few people who still remained on the island who had had a connection to his family. After a very exhaustive search, he was able to locate his nanny in her native town of Trinidad, in the central part of the island, where she was living with relatives and by then was almost blind from diabetes. The encounter engendered strong emotions and torrents of tears, and Anthony was finally able

> to thank his nanny, telling her, "You were more important to me than my own mother." He was very touched by her response, finding that she was surprised by his gratitude; she told him, "But you don't have to thank me for taking care of you, because caring for you gave me so much happiness." Anthony had always wondered if his nanny had loved him as much as he had loved her and found out the answer when she exclaimed, "Ay Tony! When you were sent away, I felt that a piece of me had been torn out. I thought I would never see you again, and I had resigned myself to live the rest of my days with that sorrow in my heart, but as of today, I can die a happy woman because I have been able to see you again."

After the trip, Anthony told his therapist that for the first time in his life he felt "complete." He began sending monetary remittances to his nanny and her family in Cuba; they maintained an active correspondence, and he visited her frequently. Then one day, he flew back to the island to attend her funeral after she died.

The personal pilgrimage in its modern secular form represents a pattern of action that can serve as an organizer to provide new integration and mastery over conflicts and to promote psychic growth. Sometimes pilgrims travel to the sites not of their own childhoods, but to the sites of their family backgrounds or of their idealized cultural origins. The pilgrim seeks to master conflicts that have been acquired by identification and to attain personal growth in the context of the person's cultural and traditional heritage; for this reason, pilgrimages are particularly important in the life stories of immigrants or their descendants. So, from a psychodynamic perspective, a pilgrimage can be conceptualized as a "flight into conflict" that leads to a new integration of the self (Poland, 1977).

REFERENCES

Beckstead, Z. (2010). Liminality in acculturation and pilgrimage: When movement becomes meaningful. *Culture and Psychology*, *16*(3), 384–393.

Duany, J. (2011). *Blurred borders: Transnational migration between the Hispanic Caribbean and the United States.* Chapel Hill: University of North Carolina Press.

Dumont, J. C., & Spielvogel. G. (2008). Return migration: A new perspective. *International Migration Outlook, 162,* 161–222. Accessed May 20, 2018. http://www.oecd.org/migration/mig/43999382.pdf

Gmelch, G. (1980). Return migration. *Annual Review of Anthropology, 9,* 135–159. Accessed May 14, 2018.

Keegan, P. J. (2017). Belonging, place, and identity: The role of social trust in developing the civic capacities of transnational Dominican youth. *High School Journal, 100*(3), 203–222. Accessed May 20, 2018.

Levitt, P. (2001). *The transnational villagers.* Berkeley: University of California Press.

Levitt, P. (2004, October 1). Transnational migrants: When "home" means more than one country. Migration Policy Institute. https://www.migrationpolicy.org/article/transnational-migrants-when-home-means-more-one-country. Accessed April 16, 2018.

Pirvu, R., & Axinte, G. (2012). Return migration: Reason, consequences and benefits. *Annals of the University of Petroșani, Economics, 12*(4), 193–202. Accessed May 20, 2018.

Poland, W. (1977). Pilgrimage: Action and tradition in self analysis. *American Journal of Psychoanalysis, 25*(2), 399–416.

Warfield, H. A., Baker, S. B., & Parikh-Foxx, S. B. (2014). The therapeutic value of pilgrimage: A grounded theory study. *Mental Health, Religion and Culture, 17*(8), 860–875. https://www.researchgate.net/publication/264901320_The_therapeutic_value_of_pilgrimage_a_grounded_theory_study. Accessed May 20, 2018.

8

Criminality Among Immigrants to the United States

Dispelling Myths and Clarifying Statistics

INTRODUCTION

National narratives portray immigrants as an essential part of American history and promote the myth of the United States as a "nation of immigrants," whereby immigrants reinforce key American values such as hard work, upward mobility, and family values (Honig, 2001). At the same time, nativist discourses also present certain immigrants as a threat to American society. This threat is both cultural, because of their presumed unwillingness or inability to assimilate, and social, because of their presumed displacement of American workers and their abuse of social services and community resources. Debates over immigration, therefore, are about not only the impact of immigrants on American society but also which immigrants are worthy or unworthy of national membership (Perea, 1997).

The discourse of immigrant criminality has been critical in constructing social boundaries throughout the history of the United States and has been prominently cited in recent immigration legislation. Yet, researchers studying the relationship between immigration and crime frequently note the discrepancy between actual rates and public perceptions of criminal behavior by immigrants. A growing body of literature shows that immigrants are less likely to engage in crime than U.S.-born citizens, and that areas with growing immigrant populations have seen decreases in crime rates. Yet, despite evidence to the contrary, public opinion surveys suggest that a large number of Americans believe that continued immigration will lead to higher levels of crime, and this is particularly true when surveys emphasize the illegal status of immigrants (Adelman, Reid, Markle, Weiss, & Jaret, 2017; Ousey & Kubrin, 2009, 2018; Passell & Cohn, 2009; Sohoni & Sohoni, 2014).

In order to better understand the debate on immigrants in crime, it is important to differentiate between the following categories that pertain to this debate (Carnegie Endowment, 1997):

1. Immigrants as criminals
2. Immigrants as crime victims
3. Terrorists who are immigrants and target the United States due to political–religious motivations
4. Organized criminal syndicates composed by immigrants, such as the Russian mafia, the South American drug cartels, people-smuggling rings, and slave prostitution rings that are run by immigrants
5. Individual immigrant felons, who commit a variety of crimes
6. Immigrant youth gangs
7. Crimes against immigrants
8. Ultimately, the sociocultural dimensions of immigrant crime

HISTORY OF IMMIGRATION AND CRIME IN THE UNITED STATES

Concerns about criminality of the foreign born were in the public debate in the United States as early as 1882, when large numbers of immigrants, predominantly from eastern Europe, began arriving on American shores. Later, in 1911, the Federal Immigration Commission, known as the Dillingham Commission, concluded that federal regulation was not effectively excluding criminal aliens and proposed strengthening the restrictions on immigration. Revisions to these laws continued in 1910 and 1917, which included laws to justify deportation. The National Origin Quota Act of 1924 began to limit and to scrutinize from which part of the world the immigrants originated and served as a criterion for admission or exclusion from the United States, partly motivated by the belief that immigrants from particular geographical origins were responsible for driving up crime rates. In the decade of the 1930s, the Commission on Law Observance and Enforcement, also known as the Wikersham Commission, devoted an entire volume to the relationship between immigration and crime but could not find a statistical connection between crimes and immigrants.

When analyzed closely, none of these investigations actually yielded any conclusive data to link immigrants to criminality. For example, the Industrial Commission of 1901, which analyzed the statistics on immigration and the foreign born, found that immigrants were actually less likely to commit crimes, but found an increase in crime among the second-generation children of immigrants, which still served as fuel against immigration. The Immigration Commission of 1911 also agreed that there was no satisfactory evidence to link immigrants and crime, and the National Commission for Law Observance of 1931 radically disagreed with the connection between immigrants and crime but did support that crime increased among the second generation. In the earlier part of the twentieth century, foreign-born individuals were more likely to be incarcerated for minor offenses such as vagrancy and drunkenness, and arrests and prosecutions for such offenses varied widely across jurisdictions and population groups. In addition, whether these offenses resulted in incarceration also depended on the economic and social resources of the offender (Moehling & Piehl, 2009).

CRIME AMONG LEGAL VERSUS UNDOCUMENTED IMMIGRANTS

It is difficult to obtain accurate statistics about crimes by immigrants due to difficulty differentiating between legal versus illegal immigrants and crimes and statistics by states because not all states keep statistics in the same manner. Immigrants who arrived legally in the United States are highly overrepresented in the incarcerated populations according to studies done in 1901, 1921, and 1931, as well as more recent studies (Clark & Anderson, 2000; Landgrave & Nowrasteh, 2017; Martinez & Lee, 2000; Motivans, 2013; Rumbaut, Gonzales, Komaie, & Morgan, 2006; Zatz & Smith, 2012). There were 39.9 million foreign-born people in the United States in 2010, and of these 44% were naturalized citizens, 24% were legal permanent residents (with a green card), and approximately 29% were unauthorized immigrants. In addition, about 3% were temporary legal residents, such as students or temporary workers. The share of the foreign-born population today is 12.9%, lower than the highest percentage of 14.8% in 1890. So, immigrants arrive largely through legal channels, but in gateway states, such as California, Texas, Arizona, New Mexico, New York, and Florida, illegal immigrants are overrepresented in the prison system, mostly due to entering the country illegally.

In 2013, there were 11.5 million undocumented immigrants living in the United States, an increase since 2011, when there were 8.5 million. Of these, 86% have been living in the United States for 7 years or longer. In 2010, about 5.2% of the labor force comprised undocumented immigrants, who comprised 3.7% of the population. Among the unauthorized immigrant population, 45% of the households were composed of couples with children. Interestingly, only 21% of U.S. native households and 34% of legal immigrant households were composed of couples with children, and by 2010, about 4.5 million U.S.-born children had at least one unauthorized immigrant parent, an increase from 2.1 million in the year 2000 (Motivans, 2013).

ILLEGAL–UNAUTHORIZED IMMIGRANTS IN THE FEDERAL, STATE, AND LOCAL JUSTICE SYSTEMS

Most of the difficulties in producing an accurate picture with regard to criminality among illegal–unauthorized immigrants stem from the fact that states have different methods of keeping crime and incarceration statistics, and there is no unified database. Also, often these databases do not differentiate whether the immigrant was incarcerated solely for entering the country illegally or for doing so in addition to other crimes (McConnell, 2013). For example, the Secure Communities Initiatives of Immigration and Customs Enforcement (ICE) 2008 revealed that the foreign-born population in the United States was about 12.5% of the total U.S. population, of which 15.3% were adults. Yet, in the total jail and prison population, foreign-born individuals represented 20%, higher than the national average. However, it is not clear how many are illegal aliens versus legal residents or citizens because they are both lumped together. It is also not clear if they were incarcerated for illegal entry, for other crimes, or for both.

In order to try to clarify some of these statistics, one should analyze the three major databases that describe crimes among illegal–unauthorized immigrants (Clark & Anderson, 2000):

1. The Pre-trial Services Act Information Systems (PSAIS), which provides information on defendants charged with federal offenses in the pretrial period

2. The United States Sentencing Commission (USSC) statistics, which provides individuals involved in the federal criminal justice system
3. The State Criminal Alien Assistance Program (SCAAP), which distributes and manages the government monies allocated for justice costs of processing and incarcerating unauthorized aliens

Pretrial Services Act Information Systems

Illegal–unauthorized aliens represented 14.4% of individuals entering the PSAIS. The number of illegal–unauthorized aliens entering the PSAIS increased by 45%, in comparison to an increase of 30% among the resident undocumented alien population. Most illegal–unauthorized aliens (60%) were charged with an immigration offense, and almost the entire increase in the number of illegal aliens entering the PSAIS can be explained by an increase in the number of illegal–unauthorized aliens arrested for immigration offenses; most of these were from California. Of those that were charged with crimes in addition to entering the United States illegally, 22% were charged with drug-trafficking offenses, compared to 50% of legal aliens and 35% of U.S. citizens. Illegal–unauthorized aliens entering the PSAIS were less educated, younger, and more likely to be White and Hispanic than legal aliens and citizens. The illegal–unauthorized aliens were more likely to be married than citizens but less likely than legal aliens (Clark & Anderson, 2000).

United States Sentencing Commission

There were 4,081 illegal–unauthorized aliens sentenced in federal district courts, 11% of the total sentenced in 1 year (1995). The number of illegal–unauthorized aliens sentenced in federal courts increased by 167%, compared with 13% for citizens. The number of legal aliens declined by 18% over same this period. The share of defendants in federal courts who were illegal–unauthorized aliens rose from 4% to 11%, while the share who were legal aliens declined from 12% to 9%. The number of illegal–unauthorized aliens sentenced increased for 89 of the 94 federal district courts for all major offense categories and for all major country of citizenship groups.

The number of illegal–unauthorized aliens appears to be partially attributable to improved border enforcement on the southwestern border. California accounted for more illegal–unauthorized aliens sentenced in federal courts than any other state, 31% of the total, followed by Texas, New York, Arizona, Florida, Oregon, and Washington. Mexicans made up the largest share of illegal aliens sentenced in federal court, followed by Colombians, Dominicans, Jamaicans, and Nigerians. Colombians were the largest group in New York, Florida, and New Jersey. Mexicans were the only group for which unlawful entry was the dominant offense. Colombians were the only group for which drug trafficking and money laundering were the dominant offenses. Nigerians were the only group for which fraud constituted a major offense.

The illegal–unauthorized aliens who were sentenced were poorer, had lower educational attainment, were younger, were more likely to be Hispanic, were more likely to be male, and were less likely to have dependents than legal aliens and citizens (Camarota & Vaughan, 2009; McConnell, 2013). Noncitizen Hispanics comprise 5.1% of the U.S. population, and of those who were sentenced for federal crimes in 2007, of all immigration offenders 74% were Hispanic. Of these, 25% were sentenced for drug trafficking, 8% for white-collar crimes, and 6% for firearms offenses (Kohut, Ketter, Doherty, Suro, & Escobar, 2006; Lopez & Livingston, 2009).

State Criminal Alien Assistance Program

According to the SCAAP database in 4 years (between 1991 and 1995), California contained a disproportionately large share of illegal alien state prisoners, 71% of the illegal aliens identified by the former Immigration and Naturalization Service (INS). The most common offenses for which illegal aliens were convicted were drug offenses in all states except Florida. For states distinguishing among types of drug offenses, drug trafficking was more common than drug possession, except in Texas. In Florida, the most common offense among illegal aliens in state prisons was murder, and both illegal and legal aliens in Florida were far more likely than aliens in other states to have been convicted of violent offenses against a person. In Florida, murder and other violent crimes were substantially more common than they were in the other major immigrant states. However, the large share of violent offenders in Florida may be an artifact related to Florida's policies of not deporting criminal aliens, which artificially increases the numbers of violent offenses of the alien criminals that are kept in the state's prisons.

Mexico was the dominant country of origin among illegal alien state prisoners, but in New York, Florida, and New Jersey, illegal immigrants from the Caribbean and from Central and South America constituted the largest shares of illegal aliens in state prisons. The vast majority of illegal alien state prisoners entered the United States illegally, rather than entering the country legally and then remaining after their authorized period of stay had expired. Colombians and Dominicans were especially likely to have been imprisoned for drug-related offenses, but among Haitians and Nicaraguans, drug offenses were relatively uncommon (Clark & Anderson, 2000; McConnell, 2013).

CRIMINALITY, IMMIGRATION, CLASS, AND RACE

Immigration, crime, and race have become intertwined in many parts of the world. In the United States, it is African Americans who have historically been a criminalized and racialized underclass, and their high rates of incarceration are one reflection of this history (Calavita, 2007). Although immigrants to the United States are feared and criminalized, their incarceration rates do not approach those of African Americans (Zatz & Smith, 2012). In the United States, Latin American illegal and legal immigrant prisoners are about 50% more likely to be incarcerated than their percentage of the population would suggest. Almost 89% of all prisoners are men; only 11.47% are women. The percentage of legal immigrant prisoners who are men or women is very similar to that of natives. However, illegal immigrant women are even less likely to be in prison than native or legal immigrant women.

In the United States, Hispanics are categorized as a single racial group in spite of the racial diversity that exists among them; they are overrepresented among the incarcerated population because they are the ones who immigrate to the United States in the largest numbers. However, when the statistics are analyzed as a whole, every group of legal and illegal immigrants, including Hispanics, has a lower incarceration rate than their native peers. Even the incarceration rate for illegal immigrants is lower than the incarceration rate for native White Americans (Stowell, Messner, McGeever, & Raffalovich, 2009).

Among those immigrants and native White Americans who are incarcerated, the great majority have lower levels of education, and individuals who have a college education among natives and among all the immigrants groups usually avoid incarceration (Kohut et al., 2006; Lopez & Livingston, 2009; Martinez & Valenzuela, 2006; Rumbaut & Ewing, 2007). A House of Representatives bill passed in December 2005 framed illegal entry into the United States as an assault against the "rule of law." Most recently, terrorism and losing control over the country's borders are mentioned in association with one another (Rumbaut et al., 2006).

When comparing the United States to other countries, in Spain and Italy the criminalization and racialization of immigrants in many ways mirror those of African Americans in the United States, and the incarceration rates of immigrants from North Africa or sub-Saharan Africa reflect this pattern (Calavita, 2005). In Europe, the overrepresentation of non-European Union (EU) citizens in prisons is between 4 and 15 times higher than for natives, higher than that of the United States. In Spain, a gateway country, the foreign prison population is 25 times higher than for natives, and most immigrants are incarcerated due to administrative violations, such as not having a residence card (Calavita, 2005). And in Italy, 25% of the prison population are immigrants, and 50% of the incarcerated minors are immigrants. In addition, most immigrants who are charged with criminal activity in Europe victimize other immigrants (Zatz & Smith, 2012).

In many other areas of law, there has been a long-standing recognition of the importance of understanding and taking into consideration the attitudes, beliefs, and values of individuals in promoting law-abiding behavior, so efforts to deter unauthorized migration through enforcement measures that ignore these underlying values are likely to be ineffective. It is important to take into account the *justificatory narratives* provided by immigrants to explain why they sometimes break the law, especially given the fact that there is an understanding and acceptance by immigrants of the racial hierarchy in the American labor market, with Whites at the top and Blacks at the bottom. For example, the immigrants emphasized their willingness to take on jobs that "not even black people want to do" (Ryo, 2015, p. 655). Their views on what is honorable and legal sometimes comes into conflict with the reality of the American labor market; "We only come to work; we don't come to harm anyone" is a common refrain among the immigrants.

In the Ryo (2015) study, immigrants were asked whether necessity justified other forms of legal noncompliance; the immigrants were unwavering in their view that crimes and other types of violations that might involve injury to third parties could not be justified even in situations of dire poverty or familial need. "These immigrants know well and beforehand that we are violating the law in crossing over without papers. But in their conscience, it's not bad because it's not a crime that they are committing. The explanation of some of the respondents was that American workers could not claim injury, as they did not want the low-wage, low-status jobs that the immigrants were willing to take" (Ryo, 2015, pp. 655–666).

CRIME IN SECOND-GENERATION IMMIGRANTS AND BEYOND

For every ethnic group without exception, the census data show an increase in rates of criminal incarceration among young men from the foreign-born to the U.S.-born generations, exactly the opposite of what is typically assumed both by standard theories and by public opinion on immigration and crime. Paradoxically, incarceration rates are lowest among immigrant young men, even among the least educated and the least acculturated among them, but they increase sharply among the U.S.-born and acculturated second generation, especially among the least educated. Children of immigrants of the second and third generations and beyond begin to show crime rates that are similar to native youth who live in socioeconomically disadvantaged areas (Rumbaut, 2004, 2005). The reasons behind the loss of protective factors of immigrants beyond the second generation are discussed elsewhere in this book.

These patterns have now been observed consistently over the last three decennial censuses, a period that covers precisely the eras of mass immigration and mass imprisonment, and they recall similar findings reported by three major commissions during the first three decades of the twentieth century, a previous era of mass migration and crime concerns, so nativity emerges in this analysis as a stronger predictor of incarceration than education (Rumbaut et al., 2006).

In Europe, by contrast, children of immigrants of the second generation and beyond show a decrease in crime rates, especially in southern Europe (Melossi, De Giorgi, & Massa, 2009). Similar findings appear in Canada (Dinovitzer, Hagan, & Levi, 2009). Some of the explanations that have been offered to explain this phenomenon include the fact that the United States has been a traditional destination for immigrants, in contrast to Europe and Canada, where the rates of immigration have increased dramatically only in recent years. It is possible that the well-established protective effect of ethnic enclaves and more sophisticated infrastructure of open communities favor early arrivals, whereas in less traditional destinations the opposite occurs. Why the second generations and beyond lose protective factors in the United States and gain them in other nontraditional destinations remains a question that merits further research (Velez & Lyons, 2012).

IMMIGRANTS AS VICTIMS

Immigrants, especially undocumented immigrants, are highly vulnerable to violence, abuse, and exploitation, and sometimes the laws and policies that are enacted in response to the fear of immigration contribute to their victimization. Illegal immigrants constitute a "shadow population" afraid to call the police or otherwise afraid to draw attention to themselves, which leaves them without protection and makes them attractive targets for victimization. These immigrants are often abused by common criminals, corrupt government officials, border vigilantes, unscrupulous employers, abusive spouses, and others. It is calculated that these undocumented immigrants are victims of at least 200,000 violent crimes and 1 million property crimes a year (Kittrie, 2006). Vulnerability may also be intensified by hostile political rhetoric aimed at increasing racialized anxiety and fear, as well as by aggressive anti-immigrant laws, and these variables are not exclusive to the United States. The metaphor of Latino immigrants "invading" the United States elicits a fear that justifies war-like strategies to defend an innocent-victim nation from a dangerous enemy (Kil & Menjívar, 2006).

Another patent example of exploitation occurs among day laborers and domestic workers. In a survey conducted among day laborers, 49% reported wage theft by employers, and 18% had been victimized by violent employers, often in the context of confrontations of work that had been completed (Valenzuela et al., 2006). This vulnerability to abuse increases among those with limited English proficiency or immigrants working in isolated conditions and when victimizers perceive that, due to a fear of deportation, the immigrant will be unlikely to report the abuse (Menjívar & Bejarano, 2004; Zatz & Smith, 2012). Due to their precarious status, many of these workers, such as janitors, gardeners, day laborers, and landscapers, often have to put in long hours and are forced to accept partial or meager payments. Female domestic workers such as maids, nannies, and caregivers who work behind the closed doors of homes have to contend with harassment and violation of labor laws and are vulnerable to sexual assault by their employers (Cepeda et al., 2012; Menjívar & Salcido, 2002).

BORDER CROSSINGS, HUMAN TRAFFICKING, VIOLENCE, AND EXPLOITATION

Border crossings across the United States–Mexico border have become increasingly more dangerous. This is partly due to the fact that policies designed to reduce the flow of immigrants into the United States have forced migrants to cross the border in remote areas where they are more likely to become lost and where the risk of death from dehydration, heat stroke, hypothermia, and drowning is heightened (McCombs, 2009). There have been an increasing number of deaths in relation to U.S. Border Patrol apprehensions. For example, the number of deaths per apprehensions across the entire border was 1.6 per 10,000 in 1999, and it increased to 7.6 per 10,000 in 2009 (Haddal, 2010) and 8.8 per 10,000 specifically in Tucson, Arizona (McCombs, 2009; Zatz & Smith, 2012). These numbers are considered to be an underestimation of the true numbers because these numbers only include the bodies that were recovered and not the skeletal remains (Haddal, 2010; Zatz & Smith, 2012).

The business of transporting persons across the border has transformed itself from small-scale smuggling operations to large trafficking schemes controlled by organized crime networks. Smuggling operations differ from human trafficking in that in smuggling, the person makes a consensual financial agreement with the smuggler or coyote, and this relationship lasts as long as the journey. Human trafficking usually involves exploitation, coercion, or deception. Victims are often crowded in large numbers into vehicles or kept in squalid conditions in drop houses during the crossing or are held hostage until a ransom is paid by family members. At other times, they are forced into indentured servitude or prostitution (Zatz & Smith, 2012).

IMMIGRATION AND NATIONAL SECURITY

After the terrorist attacks of September 11, 2001, the U.S government established the Department of Homeland Security, which represents the largest reorganization of the federal government since World War II. After more than 30 years of financial growth, the United States experienced a recession in 2008, which greatly decreased the rate of immigration from Mexico, which fell to a 40-year low in 2011. New government policies have strengthened border control of undocumented aliens, who face a greater chance of detection and removal. Between 2009 and 2015, the U.S. government removed more than 2.5 million people through immigration orders, not including the number of people who *self-deported* or were turned away or returned to their home country at the border by U.S. Customs and Border Protection.

A record high number of immigrants were ordered to be removed from the United States in 2018, a rise that many immigration advocates call the culmination of nearly 2 years of anti-immigration measures from the Trump administration. Immigration officials ordered 287,741 new deportations in the fiscal year ending September 30, 2018, and the immigration court system is heavily backlogged (Homeland Security, 2018; Smith, 2018).

In the future, the challenges that immigration represents for the United States should be met not only by effective enforcement at the borders but also by strengthening employer enforcement and better alignment with the country's labor and market needs (Meissner, Kerwin, Chishti, & Bergeron, 2013).

CONCLUSIONS

The demonization and racialization of immigrants have historically been central elements of the rhetoric surrounding U.S. immigration policy. Undocumented immigrants are portrayed as especially dangerous, sneaking into the country, committing crimes, and stealing jobs from the native born (Sohoni, 2006). However, a number of studies continue to demonstrate that immigration serves a protective function, decreasing crime rates, and that the overall crime rates are lower among immigrants than among the native born (Zatz & Smith, 2012). A recent review of 50 studies found that there was a negative correlation between immigration and crime, and that increases in the foreign-born populations in metro areas were associated with a reduction in robberies and all types of property crimes (Adelman et al., 2017).

However, studying the rates of criminality among immigrants remains a controversial issue because the data collection across the different parts of the United States is often fragmented and incomplete and because the genesis of crime involves many variables. In addition, research design varies considerably among studies (Adelman et al., 2017; Camarota & Vaughan, 2009; Ousey & Kubrin, 2018). Some of the clearer findings that emerged from the research are that immigration reduces crime in communities that have traditionally received immigrants and where ethnic enclaves with institutionalized support systems have been well established. This appears to be particularly true in urban communities where populations have declined and the arrival of immigrants has replenished and revitalized these communities.

In contrast, victimization of immigrants, especially the most vulnerable ones, such as the very poor, the low-skilled workers, and women, appears to increase in the new, nontraditional receiving communities. Here, the immigrants are prone to racialization, marginalization, and exclusion (Sampson, 2008; Zatz & Smith, 2012).

Finally, more research is needed in order to address many unanswered questions. For example, these include the contribution of post-traumatic stress disorder and crime among immigrants; the contradictions that appear when comparing American to European immigrants; the highest crime and incarceration rates among new arrivals; and the improvement of protective factors among the second-generation immigrants. Research will help to better understand the complex variables that contribute to the genesis of crime among the different nativity groups.

REFERENCES

Adelman, R., Reid, L. W., Markle, G., Weiss, S., & Jaret, C. (2017). Urban crime rates and the changing face of immigration: Evidence across four decades. *Journal of Ethnicity in Criminal Justice, 15*(1), 52–77.

Calavita, K. (2005). *Immigrants at the margins: Law, race, and exclusion in southern Europe*. Cambridge, England: Cambridge University Press.

Calavita, K. (2007). Immigration law, race, and identity. *Annual Review of Law and Social Science, 3*, 1–20.

Camarota, S. A., & Vaughan, J. M. (2009, November). Immigration and crime: Assessing a conflicted issue. Center for Immigration Studies. https://www.cis.org/sites/cis.org/files/articles/2009/crime.pdf

Carnegie Endowment. (1997). Research perspectives on migration: Immigration and the justice system, *1*(5). http://carnegieendowment.org/files/rpm/rpmvol1no5.pdf

Cepeda, A., Negi, N., Nowotny, K., Arango, J., Kaplan, C., & Valdez, A. (2012). Social stressors, special vulnerabilities and violence victimization among Latino immigrant day laborers in post Katrina New Orleans. In C. Kubrin, M. Zatz, & R. Martınez (Eds.), *Punishing immigrants: Policy, politics, and injustice* (pp. 207–231). New York: New York University Press.

Clark, R. L., & Anderson, S. A. (2000). Illegal aliens in federal, state, and local criminal justice systems. The Urban Institute. https://www.urban.org/sites/default/files/publication/62771/410366-Illegal-Aliens-in-Federal-State-and-Local-Criminal-Justice-Systems.PDF

Dinovitzer, R., Hagan, J., & Levi, R. (2009). Immigration and youthful illegalities in a global edge city. *Social* Forces, *88*, 337–372.

Haddal, C. C. (2010). Border security: The role of the U.S. Border Patrol (CRS Rep. Congr. 7-5700 RL32562). Washington, D.C.: Congressional Research Service http://www.fas.org/sgp/crs/homesec/RL32562.pdf

Homeland Security. (2018). *Yearbook of immigration statistics*. https://www.dhs.gov/immigration-statistics/yearbook. Accessed December 30, 2018.

Honig, B. (2001). *Democracy and the foreigner*. Princeton, N.J.: Princeton University Press.

Kil, S., & Menjívar, C. (2006). The "war on the border": Criminalizing immigrants and militarizing the U.S.-Mexico border. In R. Martınez & A. Valenzuela (Eds.), *Immigration and crime: Race, ethnicity and violence* (pp. 164–188). New York: New York University Press.

Kittrie, O. (2006). Federalism, deportation, and crime victims afraid to call the police. *Iowa Law Review, 91*, 1449–1508.

Kohut, A., Ketter, S., Doherty, C., Suro, R., & Escobar, G. (2006). America's immigration quandary. Report prepared by the Pew Research Center for the People & the Press and the Pew Hispanic Center. https://www.pewresearch.org/hispanic/2006/03/30/americas-immigration-quandary/

Landgrave, M., & Nowrasteh, A. (2017). Criminal immigrants: Their numbers, demographics, and countries of origin *Immigration and Research Policy Brief,*

March 15, *1*. https://www.cato.org/publications/immigration-reform-bulletin/criminal-immigrants-their-numbers-demographics-countries

Lopez, M. H., & Livingston, G. (2009, April 7). Hispanics and the criminal justice system: Low confidence, high exposure. Pew Hispanic Trust. http://www.pewhispanic.org/files/reports/106.pdf

Martinez, R., & Lee, M. T. (2000). On immigration and crime. The nature of crime: Continuity and change. *Criminal Justice*, *1*, 485–524. https://www.ncjrs.gov/criminal_justice2000/vol_1/02j.pdf

Martinez, R., & Valenzuela, A. (2006). *Immigration and crime: Race, ethnicity and violence*. New York: New York University Press.

McCombs, B. (2009, December 27). No signs of letup in entrant deaths. *Arizona Daily Star*. http://azstarnet.com/news/local/border/article_faf5b437-b728-527b-9eb8-77977d0cdf84.html

McConnell, E. H. (2013). Illegal immigrants and corrections. In J. S. Albanese (Ed.), *The encyclopedia of criminology and criminal justice* (pp. 1–3). New York: Wiley. https://onlinelibrary.wiley.com/doi/10.1002/9781118517383.wbeccj081

Meissner, D., Kerwin, D. M., Chishti, M., & Bergeron, C. (2013). Immigration enforcement in the United States: The rise of a formidable machinery. Migration Policy Institute. https://www.migrationpolicy.org/research/immigration-enforcement-united-states-rise-formidable-machinery. Accessed December 28, 2018.

Melossi, D., De Giorgi, A., & Massa, E. (2009). The "normality" of "'second generations" in Italy and the importance of legal status: A self-report delinquency study. In W. McDonald (Ed.), *Immigration, crime and justice* (pp. 47–65). New York: Emerald.

Menjívar, C., & Bejarano, C. (2004). Latino immigrants' perceptions of crime and police authorities in the United States: A case study from the Phoenix metropolitan area. *Ethnic and Racial Studies*, *27*, 120–148.

Menjívar, C., & Salcido, O. (2002). Immigrant women and domestic violence: Common experiences in different countries. *Gender & Society*, *15*, 898–920.

Moehling, C., & Piehl, A. M. (2009). Immigration, crime, and incarceration in early twentieth-century America. *Demography*, *46*(4), 739–763. http://europepmc.org/articles/PMC2831353

Motivans, M. (2013, October 22). Federal Justice Statistics Program: Immigration offenders in the federal justice system in 2010. https://www.bjs.gov/content/pub/pdf/iofjs10.pdf

Ousey, G., & Kubrin, C. (2009). Exploring the connection between immigration and violent crime rates in U.S. cities, 1980–2000. *Social Problems*, *56*, 447–473.

Ousey, G., & Kubrin, C. (2018). Immigration and crime: Assessing a contentious issue. *Annual Review of Criminology*, *1*(1), 63–84. http://www.annualreviews.org/doi/abs/10.1146/annurev-criminol-032317-092026. Accessed January 7, 2018.

Passell, J., & Cohn, D. (2009). *A portrait of unauthorized immigrants in the United States*. Washington, D.C.: Pew Research Center. http://pewresearch.org/pubs/1190/portrait-unauthorized-immigrants-states

Perea, J. F. (1997). *Immigrants out! The new nativism and the anti-immigrant impulse in the United States*. New York: New York University Press.

Rumbaut, R. G. (2004). Ages, life stages, and generational cohorts: Decomposing the immigrant first and second generations in the United States. *International Migration Review, 38*(3), 1160–1205.

Rumbaut, R. G. (2005). Turning points in the transition to adulthood: Determinants of educational attainment, incarceration, and early childbearing among children of immigrants. *Ethnic and Racial Studies, 28*(6), 1041–1086.

Rumbaut, R. G., & Ewing, W. (2007). *The myth of immigrant criminality and the paradox of assimilation: Incarceration rates among native and foreign-born men.* Washington, D.C.: American Immigration Law Foundation.

Rumbaut, R. G., Gonzales, R. G., Komaie, G., & Morgan, C. V. (2006, June 1). Debunking the myth of immigrant criminality: Imprisonment among first and second-generation young men. Migration Policy Institute. https://www.migrationpolicy.org/article/debunking-myth-immigrant-criminality-imprisonment-among-first-and-second-generation-young/

Ryo, E. (2015). Less enforcement, more compliance: Rethinking unauthorized migration. *UCLA Law Review, 62*, 622–670.

Sampson, R. (2008). Rethinking crime and immigration. *Contexts, 7*, 28–33.

Smith, K. (2018, November 8). Immigrant deportation filings hit record high in 2018, new report shows. *CBS News.* https://www.cbsnews.com/news/ice-deportations-in-2018-hit-record-high/. Accessed December 30, 2018.

Sohoni, D. (2006). The immigrant problem: Modern day nativism on the web. *Current Sociology, 54*, 827–850.

Sohoni, D., & Sohoni, T. W. P. (2014). Perceptions of immigrant criminality: Crime and social boundaries. *The Sociological Quarterly, 55*, 49–71.

Stowell, J., Messner, S., McGeever, K., & Raffalovich, L. (2009). Immigration and the recent violent crime drop in the United States: A pooled, cross-sectional time-series analysis of metropolitan areas. *Criminology, 47*, 889–928.

Valenzuela, A., Theodore, N., Melendez, E., & Gonzalez, A. (2006). *On the Corner: Day Labor in the U.S.* Los Angeles: University of California, Los Angeles Center Study Urban Poverty.

Velez, M., & Lyons, C. (2012). Situating the immigration and neighborhood crime relationship across multiple cities. In C. Kubrin, M. Zatz, & R. Martınez (Eds.), *Punishing immigrants: Policy, politics, and injustice* (pp. 159–177). New York: New York University Press.

Zatz, M. S., & Smith, H. (2012). Immigration, crime and victimization: Rhetoric and reality. *Annual Review of Law and Social Science, 8*, 141–159.

9

The Immigrant Narrative

Life stories sometimes say as much about the culture wherein they are told as they do about the teller of the story. McAdams (2006) has studied the characteristics of the national American narrative, which he has called *the redemptive self*. He explained that for the past 200 years immigrants arriving in the United States have traditionally subscribed to this narrative in order to describe their experience of migration, arrival, and acculturation into the American mainstream. People typically use stories to describe how the world works and why and how human beings do what they do. A person's life story is an internalized, evolving narrative of the self that provides life with some degree of coherence. It weaves together the reconstructed past, the perceived present, and the anticipated future in an effort to provide the self with a feeling of purpose and unity (McAdams, 2001).

This life story model suggests that narrative is also a means of identity development, and that individuals construct their lives as evolving stories. According to this model, people can have many narrative identities, and storytelling can help integrate the conflicting narratives into a single narrative identity and, in turn, support a coherent sense of self and affirm life's meaning and purpose (McAdams, 2008).

The role of narrative as a characteristic form of psychodynamic and psychoanalytic explanation has also become increasingly common, and the construction of narrative in the clinical encounter is now becoming recognized as an important therapeutic tool. Spence (1982) has written about the differences between *historical truth* and *narrative truth*. He explained that historical truth refers to the aim of the narrator to come as close as possible to what really happened in the original event. In contrast, narrative truth is an attempt at interpreting and understanding the memory of the event with the conviction that the interpretation given by the narrator must be true. Narrative truth is also an attempt at using language to capture complex images and emotions in the form of a cohesive story that can be more easily understood (Howard, 1991).

This chapter addresses the importance of the immigrant narrative from a psychodynamic and developmental perspective. It explains how narratives can serve as a useful therapeutic tool to help the immigrant work through the traumas and losses associated with migration and to negotiate the different stages of transformation of the immigrant's identity that often result from the process of acculturation. Finally, this chapter also addresses the role of the narrative as an important tool for psychological growth.

THE AMERICAN NARRATIVE

Erikson (1950/1993) explained that *generativity* constituted the most important accomplishment of adult life. Starting in adolescence, people begin to generate particular narratives that help them attain positive functioning in many aspects of their lives, to broaden their social networks and attachments and face the daunting challenges of midlife. These narratives frequently focus on the important chapters of a person's life—the low points, high points, and turning points; their hopes and plans for the future—as well as attach meaning to the person's life journey. People's life stories are largely drawn from a menu of available story options provided by their culture. These menus provide the necessary structure for individual storytelling. Stories are collaborative endeavors, coconstructed in the real or imagined act of being told, so the listener and the culture where the story is being told have a strong influence in shaping the story. These influences have been well documented. In the case of the American narrative and other national or regional narratives, these social and cultural influences can sometimes prove oppressive to people whose lives do not easily conform to dominant cultural plots or themes that are accepted or demanded by the host culture or by the dominant majority.

McAdams (2001, 2006, 2008) postulated that there is a distinct *American narrative* that is also closely tied to the *American immigrant narrative.* He argued that this narrative can be traced back to Puritan autobiographies and can be seen in many American novels and Hollywood movies in which highly generative men and women tell stories that emphasize themes of suffering, redemption, and personal destiny. He has called it the redemptive self.

The most representative of these stories are those written by Horatio Alger (1832–1899), the well-known nineteenth-century American writer who depicted the lives of young adults and their rise from humble backgrounds to lives of middle-class security and comfort through hard work, determination, courage, and honesty. His writings exemplified the *Protestant work ethic* and were characterized by the narrative, which had a formative effect on America during the Gilded Age (McGlinn, 2004). This *redemptive narrative* focuses on moving from a negative to a positive situation and outlines the sequence of events in the creation of the redemptive self. The redemptive narrative begins with (1) a person who enjoys a special advantage, (2) who suffered injustice in his or her life or witnessed it in the life of others, (3) who begins to consolidate a sense of moral steadfastness by the end of adolescence and, (4) after encountering negative events, he or she transforms these into redemptive events, and (5) as he or she moves ahead in life, sets pro-social goals aimed at improving the life of others and leaving a legacy of him- or herself. The redemptive self not only is a quintessentially American identity but also represents the quintessentially American immigrant identity (McAdams, 2012; Singer, 2004). Cushman (1995) has argued that this very American metaphor for understanding the inner self, the *human interior*, mirrors the American sense of geography. Like the heartland of North America, the inner self is large and good, and it is our manifest destiny to liberate it, to free up and actualize its vast potential.

McAdams's research showed that highly generative adults are five times more likely than less generative adults to import spontaneously into their life narrative accounts a discrete childhood incident in which they felt empathy for the suffering of another or witnessed an injustice experienced by another person. It is as if these narrators want their listeners to know this about the beginnings of their stories: I was blessed, but others suffered, or to put it differently, I was chosen for a special destiny in a dangerous world.

The redemptive self provides Americans of many different persuasions, as well as immigrants to America, with a common language or format for making sense of an individual life. The way the story plays out is that bad things often lead to good outcomes, and my suffering is redeemed because suffering can be overcome and redemption typically follows life's setbacks and failures. Redemption comes to me in the form of atonement, recovery, emancipation, enlightenment, upward social mobility, or the actualization of my good inner self. As the plot unfolds, I continue to grow and progress. I bear fruit; I give back; I offer a unique contribution. I will make a happy ending, even in a threatening world.

Some of these points are clearly illustrated by the narrative of Rosileidy, a 29-year-old Cuban American female social worker who in 1994, at the age of 9, fled the island of Cuba with her parents on a raft. In the midst of a very dangerous sea voyage, the family was intercepted at sea by the U.S. Coast Guard and confined for 5 months to a refugee camp prior to arriving in the United States. This is how she narrated her story:

Case I

> When my parents boarded us on that raft to bring us here, they gambled against death. We were all very lucky that they won that hand. Now that I am going to be a mother, I have often wondered if I would have the courage to do the same thing for my child. All I can say is that I hope life never puts me in that kind of situation. When I think about how it was that I got to this country, I feel a deep sense of responsibility. I tell myself that I must always try "to be the best that I can be," as a mother, as a wife, and as a professional because that was the reason for my parents sacrifice.

The American narrative of the redemptive self has often been criticized for being simplistic and naïve and for ignoring the tragedies of life. Tragedy gives a fuller expression to the ambivalence and multiplicity of the human factors that are involved in life outcomes. The tragic hero learns that suffering is an essential part of human life, and that often suffering has no ultimate meaning, benefit, or human cause and that suffering is to be endured, but not necessarily redeemed. The hero learns that human beings are moral agents, but that not every action or event makes sense in a moral framework. Tragedy teaches us that sometimes the individual is not responsible for his or her fate, and that sometimes fate cannot be avoided. The redemptive self celebrates the power of resilience and growth, but it may also fall prey to arrogance and self-righteousness.

MEMORY AND THE NARRATIVE

It is important to understand some concepts about the neurophysiology of memory in order to understand how narratives are constructed. As early as 1937, Freud (1937/1964) questioned the veracity and accuracy of recovered memories and recognized the limitations of remembering events exactly how they occurred. New advances in neurophysiology have shed light on how human memories are encoded. *Semantic* or *declarative* memory is an active verbal constructive process that takes place once the frontal lobe and neocortex areas have been engaged. Semantic or declarative memory creates a verbal description of preexisting mental *schemata*. A *schema* is a pattern of thought and behavior that organizes categories of information and the relationships among them, a process that occurs predominantly in the limbic system, a more primitive and nonverbal part of the brain.

The parts of the brain responsible for semantic–declarative memory do not become myelinated until the fourth year of life, which is why memories that occur prior to this period are stored as a *sensorimotor, nonverbal* experience. Most memory storage involves only the limbic system and does not engage the frontal lobe and the neocortex, so most of the processing of memories occurs outside conscious awareness. Only novel stimuli are processed through the frontal lobe and the neocortex as a new experience worth being noted. The *amygdalas*, located in the limbic system, evaluate the emotional state of the person that was produced by an event and assign emotional meaning to the experience. Another structure in the limbic system, the *septohippocampal system*, evaluates temporally and spatially unrelated events and connects how they are related to each other. So, in essence, it can be said that memories of important events are encoded in the brain as a series of complex visual images that have an affective component attached to them. These memories are also organized in time and space with relation to other previously encoded memories (Eid, Johnsen, & Saus, 2005).

NORMAL AND TRAUMATIC DISTORTIONS OF MEMORY

The process of encoding a memory into the brain can be conceptualized as the first translation of an event that occurred in reality. Later, an attempt at putting that memory into words can be considered as a second translation of the original event. The complexity of the event and the impact the event may have had on the observer are very difficult to capture in words, so the narrative account of the memory of an event is a creative exercise that will yield a somewhat different product than what occurred in reality.

Ultimately, the interaction and dialogue with the listener, in some cases the therapist, also distort and alter the recollection of the event. In the case of trauma, increased arousal produces an increase in norepinephrine in the brain. While moderately high levels of arousal may increase curiosity and novelty seeking, very high levels of arousal produce fear and cause the individual to avoid novelty seeking and to perseverate on familiar behaviors, regardless of the outcome. This physiological mechanism may explain the classical defense mechanism of *repetition–compulsion* that is associated with trauma, as well as the obsessive and avoidant behaviors that are frequently associated with *post-traumatic stress disorder* (PTSD).

Increased norepinephrine interferes with the consolidation of semantic–declarative memory by causing the amygdalas to override the frontal lobe and the neocortex, producing a *sensorimotor memory* devoid of a narrative. In addition, elevated levels of the stress hormone *cortisol* produce a decrease of activity in the septohippocampal system, which causes an inability to categorize the memory in a symbolic form and in relation to other schemas or to remember the event in time and space.

The release of stress hormones in new situations of stress and danger may reactivate visual images of the trauma that appear in the form of *flashbacks*. These *sensorimotor, nondeclarative* memories that are caused by trauma are produced when there is a hyperarousal of the amygdala and a shutdown of the septohippocampal system and become indelible and devoid of a narrative (Leyton & Krikorian, 2002; Van der Kolk, 2003). Many immigrants suffer multiple separations from loved ones, massive human and material losses, and various degrees of trauma in the process of migration and acculturation. PTSD occurs when individuals process trauma in a way that leads to a sense of ongoing, serious threat. Individuals who have participated in, or who have been victims of, acts of cruelty and inhumanity continue to experience these memories and to live in an internal context of inhumanity long after the events have ended and the survivor is left with a central schema and a personal narrative that is defined by trauma (Bohlinger, 2010). In addition to the sense of ever-present threat, these individuals experience a sense of a foreshortened future.

Psychologically traumatized individuals develop embedded negative appraisals of what will happen to them in the future. This results from the natural protective mechanism of avoidant behavior, which appears when human beings are faced with adverse and catastrophic events (Horowitz, 2011). Avoidance also interferes with the capacity of the individual to elaborate and contextualize a detailed narrative of what occurred, and lacking a narrative, the person is unable to assimilate the complete traumatic event.

Some individuals encounter difficulties producing a coherent and significant story and remain with only a partial story of the trauma. Research has demonstrated that these individuals are more prone to developing PTSD (Pennebaker & Seagal, 1999; Van Minnen, Wessel, Dikjstra, & Roelofs, 2002; Wrigen, 1994; Zoellner, Alvarez-Conrad, & Foa, 2002). Some of these concepts are illustrated by the case of Mrs. Restrepo, a 54-year-old South American woman who arrived in the United States with her husband and three children after the release of her 21-year-old daughter, who had been kidnapped and held captive for more than a year by a guerrilla group in her country of origin. The husband sold his business and declared bankruptcy in order to pay the elevated ransom necessary to recover their daughter. Mrs. Restrepo explained her emotional state to the therapist in the following way:

CASE II

> For more than a year, we lived in a panic that our daughter could be murdered by the "Guerrillas." During that time, my husband and I constantly told each other that we needed to suppress all our emotions and to be cool, to not do anything impulsive that would provoke our daughter's captors or to make a mistake that could cost our daughter her life. Now, when I try to remember that period of time, it seems to me like I was living in a dream, as if all of that had happened to somebody else and I can't seem to remember any

> of the details. I felt that during that time I was functioning like a robot. Now we've been in the U.S. for more than a year and I will not let my daughter out of my sight. We hardly go outside, and we are always together. Strangely, I continue to live with a constant fear that if I allow myself to be angry at my daughter's captors, they could still somehow take her away from me and kill her.

People who suffer from PTSD will process trauma in a way that leads to a sense of serious and current threat. Negative appraisals of the trauma are fueled by poor elaborations of the narrative of the traumatic events, which are prevented into developing into full elaborations due to the avoidant behavior. In these survivors, high levels of post-traumatic symptoms are seen to emerge over time and further interfere with the capacity to assimilate the traumatic event by increasing avoidance. This avoidance sometimes begins immediately after the traumatic event in the form of a *peritraumatic dissociation*, which interferes with the encoding of memories and leads to incomplete and fragmented narratives that are devoid of meaning (Amir, Stafford, Freshman, & Foa, 1998; Gidron et al., 2002).

This mechanism of avoidance and fixation on a negative appraisal of the future is illustrated in the narrative of Julian, a 66-year-old Cuban American man who left Cuba as an "unaccompanied minor" after his parents sent him to the United States in order to avoid forced conscription by the government into a communist boarding school. He described his departure in the following terms:

CASE III

> I remember seeing my mother's face through the glass wall of the waiting room in the airport in Havana, a place that they called "the fishbowl." There were many people there that day and a lot of chaos, and she was trying to tell us something, but we couldn't hear anything through the glass enclosure. I was clutching my sister's hand, and I was so scared. It's funny because I can't remember anything else

> that happened afterward on that day or for the following weeks and months. We were finally able to reunite with my mother in the U.S. a year and a half later, but everyone else that I loved and everything that was dear to me was left behind on that day. I was 11 years old at the time, and since then I have always felt that anything that is good in my life, or any person that I love, will only be a part of my life for a little while and that soon afterward I am destined to lose them.

THE HEALING EFFECT OF THE IMMIGRANT'S LIFE NARRATIVE

The life story shapes and influences the identity of the narrator. Individuals who have been traumatized perceive the world as less safe, have a lower sense of self-worth, and find less meaning in the world. The psychologically healthy individual is one who is capable of holding a (1) coherent, (2) dynamic, and (3) meaningful narrative of the self. The development of a person's identity also involves an exercise of life story construction, so psychopathology can be seen as "life stories gone awry." Psychotherapy, which involves the reconstruction of the life narrative, can then be seen as "an exercise of life story repair." Trauma, by definition, breaks the smooth progression of daily life and its continuity. It disrupts the narrative process at two levels, (1) the narrative of the specific traumatic event and (2) the entire life story of the individual (Wrigen, 1994).

In psychotherapy, the therapist and the patient work jointly at creating an alternative story, which is richer and one in which identity is promoted. The goal of creating a trauma narrative, which will become the patient's narrative truth, needs to have three elements: (1) continuity and coherence, (2) self-evaluation, and (3) the creation of meaning. Later, narratives about the psychotherapy enable the patient to remember the lessons learned during the work of therapy.

Immigrants and the children of immigrants can construct narratives in an internal dialogue with themselves or in conversation with members of their family or community. These narratives are re-edited and enriched by the narrator with the passage of time and with the acquisition of maturity, wisdom, and experience. They will also allow the individual to continue an active process of ongoing psychological growth by way of introspection and self-exploration (Adler, Wagner, & McAdams, 2007; Spence, 1982).

In the case of traumatized persons, creating a trauma story through information, construction, and cognitive processing helps the individual charge the event with personal meaning and to place it as a part of the rest of his or her life, rather than it being the central focus of the person's life. The context of the trauma story will take place in three spheres of context: (1) *the intersubjective or interpersonal context*, which includes the relations and interactions of the narrator and its interlocutors and how the story affects both; (2) *the social field*, which includes the persons, organizations, and particular time in which the story occurred; and 3) *the cultural metanarratives,* which refer to the relation of the individual's personal story in relation to the historical and political events that coincide with the times in which the story is taking place and which will imbue the story with particular interpretations. They also describe the culture's expectations about how lives are to be lived (Zilber, Tuval-Mashiach, & Lieblich, 2008).

Coherence in the narrative is deeply influenced by the temperament, personality, and level of ego development of the narrator. Individuals with a temperamental inclination to neuroticism, for instance, have been found to produce life stories that emphasize bad outcomes, depression, low self-esteem, and more life dissatisfaction. Immature individuals with low levels of ego development tend to relate simplistic life stories, which are conventional, seek stability, and avoid change, including growth. They tend to lack meaning, purpose, and a sense of future direction. In contrast, individuals with more mature ego development describe richer life stories and are able to integrate complex, often contradictory, aspects of an event (Amir et al., 1998; Pennebaker & Seagal, 1999; Tuval-Mashiach et al., 2004; Van Minnen et al., 2002; Zoellner et al., 2002). Such is the case of Alberto, who arrived in the United States as a political refugee at the age to 28 after having served 6 years in a Communist political prison for opposing the government of his country of origin. He narrated the following:

CASE IV

> Everyone I knew growing up had already left my country. I stayed behind because I was young and naïve and idealistic, and I thought I should fight against a political system that had been forcefully imposed on my country and which I believed was unfair and oppressive. I paid a high price by losing 6 years of my life, but I feel fortunate that I made it out alive. When I was in prison, we heard gunshots every day at 5 in the morning. It was because my fellow prisoners were being executed by the firing squads. I lived in terror waiting for the day my name would be called next. Most of what went on in prison I can barely remember. It's as if it was all part of a nightmare. One day they called my name, and I thought I was going to be executed. Instead, they ordered me to take off my prisoner's uniform, they gave me some civilian clothes to wear, and they told me I was going to the airport. I still thought it was a cynical joke and that I was going to be driven to some faraway place to be executed, but I breathed a sigh of relief when the airplane took off and I saw my country receding in the distance. I ended up in Newark, New Jersey, working in a factory. My arrival there coincided with the city going up in flames during the riots that followed the death of Martin Luther King. I felt so scared during that time that I can swear to you, at times I fantasized about returning back to my former prison cell in search of safety. I felt a great sense of desolation during those first years in the United States. I felt that no one would be able to understand what I had gone through and kept everything to myself. At the time, I was having anxiety attacks, and I had a repetitive dream in which I saw a pendulum of a clock swinging from left to right. At one end was the face of my mother and in the other end was the face of my nanny, the two people I have loved the most in my life. I had

> that dream over and over for years. It was my wife, who is American, who dragged me to see a psychiatrist after we got married because she was concerned about me. For the first time, I was able to tell my story and to feel understood, and I realized that everything I was feeling was normal, given the experiences I had been through. I was able to start life anew, and very slowly the pervasive sadness that followed me everywhere began to subside. Now I have five wonderful children and already two grandchildren, I love this country, I have risen to a high managerial position, I have a successful career, and I feel very American. Where else in the world can one be able to tell such a story?

One of the most common features found among the people who have been psychologically traumatized is a pervasive sense of "existential loneliness" based on the feeling that "only someone who has been through what I have been through would be able to understand." These feelings of emotional and social isolation may ultimately lead to depression and substance abuse. For these victims, who often long for empathy and understanding from others, the creation of a narrative can also serve as a vehicle of communication that can (1) enhance a feeling of communion with others, (2) enhance a sense of agency and self-efficacy, and (3) help the person redefine his or her ultimate life concerns, such as ethical, moral, spiritual, and religious goals and values (Stein & Tuval-Mashiach, 2014).

THE IMMIGRANT NARRATIVE IN CONTEMPORARY LITERATURE

Literary fiction with young adult immigrant protagonists is an important vehicle to understand the realities of these new generations of Americans. Clifford and Kalyanpur (2011) studied 20 young adult novels published since 2000 that narrated the immigrant experience. They analyzed these narratives taking into account (1) the experiences prior to migration; (2) the journeys of immigration; (3) the experiences and adjustments of arriving in the host country; and (4) the dynamics of power. These narratives, which encompass works of fiction, biography, and historical novels, focused on the poverty, discrimination, and violence in the immigrant's homeland prior to departure and on the sometimes-unrealistic dreams of finding a different reality in America. These accounts are followed by difficult journeys by boat, by train, on foot, or by mule and encountering dangerous conditions, exploitation, and abuse along the way and difficult and perilous encounters with immigration officials. Once these immigrants arrive in the United States, there is a clash of cultures and massive adjustments, which are particularly hard for teenagers and which are discussed in other chapters of this book. The dynamics of power also play an important role in these novels, with the acquisition of nonaccented English and often the Americanization of the person's name as landmarks of successful acculturation and protection against discrimination and marginalization. The dynamics of race and class are closely related to themes of power, and the accentuation of differences between the immigrant and the members of the host culture is regarded as a *deficit* that needs to be overcome. These authors suggested that teachers would do well in exposing immigrants and native-born students to these literary immigrant narratives in order to widen their understanding of their own lives and the lives of others and to help build a more accepting and harmonious society.

CONCLUSIONS

The immigrant experience is one of the most stressful experiences a person can undergo. It removes the immigrants from their relationships, friends, neighbors, and members of the extended family. It also removes the immigrants from their community, jobs, customs, and sometimes language, placing them in a strange and unpredictable environment (Ticho, 1971). Narratives are important to all human beings, but particularly in the case of immigrants, the creation of narratives gives shape to events and allows for the integration and understanding of previously challenging and troubling experiences. It creates a *new paradigm shift* where (1) the world is seen from a new perspective and where (2) new options appear and (3) new actions become possible.

The effort of creating a narrative is not toward describing the inexhaustible complexity of invisible facts, but at turning them into something that is simple and visible (Roth, 1991). As the person traverses the different stages of his or her life, narratives will be constantly revisited and re-edited to reflect the different perspective that is characteristic of the person's particular life stage. The immigrant narrative can help these individuals to restructure their life stories, to reorganize meaning, to suggest purpose, and to foreshadow where the person's life story is headed. They also allow immigrants to reclaim competency, recognize resiliency in themselves, and move into a positive and life-affirming direction.

REFERENCES

Adler, J. M., Wagner, J. W., & McAdams, D. P. (2007). Personality and the coherence of psychotherapy narratives. *Journal of Research in Personality, 41*, 1179–1198.

Amir, N., Stafford, J., Freshman, M. S., & Foa, E. B. (1998). Relationship between trauma narratives and trauma pathology. *Journal of Traumatic Stress, 11*, 385–392.

Bohlinger, A. (2010). *Post-traumatic stress disorder and narrative therapy* (Dissertation, University of Wisconsin, Stout). http://annaboh.files.wordpress.com/2010/06/narrative-therapy-ptsd.pdf. Accessed March 4, 2018.

Clifford, E., & Kalyanpur, M. (2011). Immigrant narratives: Power, difference, and representation in young-adult novels with immigrant protagonists. *International Journal of Multicultural Education, 13*(1). https://files.eric.ed.gov/fulltext/EJ1109701.pdf. Accessed March 1, 2018.

Cushman, P. (1995). *Constructing the self, constructing America: A cultural history of psychotherapy.* Reading, MA: Addison-Wesley.

Eid, J., Johnsen, B. H., & Saus, E. R. (2005). Trauma narrative and emotional processing. *Scandinavian Journal of Psychology, 46*, 503–510.

Erikson, E. H. (1950/1993). *Childhood and Society*. New York: Norton.

Freud, S. (1964). *Constructions in analysis*. Standard edition, Vol. *23*. London: Hogarth Press. (Original work published 1937)

Gidron, Y., Duncan, E., Lazar, A., Biderman, A., Tandeter, H., & Schwartzman, P. (2002). Effects of guided written disclosure of stressful experiences on clinic visits and symptoms in frequent clinic attenders. *Family Practice, 19*, 161–166.

Horowitz, M. (2011). *The stress response syndromes: PTSD, grief, adjustment and dissociative disorder.* 5th ed. Lanham, MD: Aronson.

Howard, G. S. (1991). Cultural tales: A narrative approach to thinking, cross-cultural psychology and psychotherapy. *American Psychologist, 46*, 187–197.

Leyton, B., & Krikorian, R. (2002). Memory mechanisms in post-traumatic stress disorder. *Journal of Neuropsychiatry and Clinical Neurosciences, 14*, 254–261.

McAdams, D. P. (2001). The psychology of life stories. *Review of General Psychology, 5*, 100–122.

McAdams, D. P. (2006). *The redemptive self: Stories Americans live by*. New York: Oxford University Press.

McAdams, D. P. (2008). Personal narratives and the life story. In O. P. John, R. W. Robins, & L.A. Pervin (Eds.), *Handbook of personality theory and research* (3rd ed., pp. 100–122). New York: Guilford Press.

McAdams, D. P. (2012). Exploring psychological themes through life-narrative accounts. In J. A. Holstein & J. F. Gubrium (Eds.), *Varieties of narrative analysis* (pp. 15–32). Thousand Oaks, CA: Safe Publications.

McGlinn, J. (2004). Rags to riches: The Horatio Alger theme in adolescent novels about the immigrant experience. *The Allan Review, 34*(3). Virginia Technological University. http://scholar.lib.vt.edu/ejournals/ALAN/v31n3/mcglinn.html. Accessed February 24, 2018.

Pennebaker, J. W., & Seagal, J. D. (1999). Forming a story: Health benefits of narrative. *Journal of Clinical Psychology, 55*(10), 1243–1254.

Roth, P. (1991). Truth in interpretation: The case of psychoanalysis. *Philosophy of the Social Sciences, 21*, 175–195.

Singer, J. A. (2004). Narrative identity and narrative meaning across the life-span. *Journal of Personality, 72*(3), 437–459.

Spence, D. P. (1982). *Narrative truth and historical truth: Meaning and interpretation in psychoanalysis*. New York: Norton.

Stein, J. Y., & Tuval-Mashiash, R. (2014). Loneliness and isolation in life-stories of Israeli veterans of combat and captivity. *Psychological Trauma Theory Research Practice and Policy*. https://www.researchgate.net/publication/262639083_Loneliness_and_Isolation_in_Life-Stories_of_Israeli_Veterans_of_Combat_and_Captivity. Accessed March 4, 2018.

Ticho, G. (1971). Cultural aspects of transference and countertransference. *Bulletin of the Menninger Clinic, 35*, 313–326.

Tuval-Mashiach, R., Freedman, S., Bargai, N., Boker, R., Hadar, H., & Shalev A. Y. (2004). Coping with trauma: Narrative and cognitive perspectives. *Psychiatry, 67*(3), 280–293.

Van der Kolk, B. (2003). The neurobiology of childhood trauma and abuse. *Child and Adolescent Psychiatric Clinics of North America, 12*, 296–317.

Van Minnen, A., Wessel, I., Dikjstra T., & Roelofs, K. (2002). Changes in PTSD patient narratives during prolonged exposure therapy: A replication and extension. *Journal of Traumatic Stress, 15*, 255–258.

Wrigen, J. (1994). Narrative completion in the treatment of trauma. *Psychotherapy Theory, Research, Practice, Training, 31*(3), 414–423.

Zilber, T. M., Tuval-Mashiach, R., & Lieblich, A. (2008). The embedded narrative: Navigating through multiple contexts. *Qualitative Inquiry, 14*, 1047–1069.

Zoellner, L., Alvarez-Conrad, J., & Foa, E. (2002). Peritraumatic dissociative experiences, trauma narratives, and trauma pathology. *Journal of Traumatic Stress, 15*(1), 49–57.

10

Treatment Interventions for Immigrants, Refugees, and Their Families

Immigrants and refugees are becoming a growing segment of the demographics of the United States, reaching 18.8% or 78.2 million by 2060. It is a segment that is culturally more diverse than the U.S.-born population (Colby & Ortman, 2015). This is as a result of not only the progressive aging and low birth rate of the European-origin population and the significant rise in immigration from non-European countries, especially from Latin America, Asia, and Africa. Therefore, there is a growing demand for the provision of appropriate and effective mental health services for immigrants and refugees, now representing a larger segment of the overall population. At the same time, the process of evaluating and treating culturally diverse immigrants and their families can be complex and requires unique approaches, most of these related to the diversity in cultures and cultural values as well as the unique stressful experiences these populations have undergone.

PRINCIPLES AND DEFINITIONS

We first define the principles and concepts we believe undergird the approaches to the mental health treatment of immigrants and refugees, then follow with a model for their application as well as examples of interventions that have demonstrated beginning evidence.

The cultural competence model. The cultural competence model for mental health services is a key to serving immigrants and refugees. *Cultural competence* is a set of congruent behaviors, attitudes, and policies found in systems, agencies, or individual professionals that enables them to work effectively in a context of cultural difference (Cross, Bazron, Dennis, & Isaacs, 1989). In response to these mounting clinical and service delivery challenges, cultural competence became one of the core principles of the children's community-based systems of care movement from its outset given the rapidly growing populations of culturally diverse children in the United States and their unmet mental health needs. Cross and colleagues identified a spectrum of cultural competence that has been demonstrated by societies and their institutions over centuries, ranging from cultural destructiveness (genocide, lynching, ethnic cleansing); cultural incapacity (segregation, discrimination, immigration quotas, services that break up families); cultural blindness ("equal" treatment for all, but not making distinctions in services offered on differences in values or beliefs); cultural precompetency (realization of differences but insufficient provision of services); to cultural competence. Few societies have achieved the last stage, cultural proficiency (provision of innovative, culturally specific services and research). They went on to define characteristics that culturally competent clinicians and organizations represented. For clinicians, they cited the key elements of awareness/acceptance of difference, awareness of own cultural values, understanding dynamics of difference in the clinical encounter, the development of clinically relevant cultural knowledge, and the ability to adapt practice to the cultural context of the patient. For the organization, they cited valuing diversity, the performance of cultural self-assessments, management of the dynamics of difference, institutionalization of cultural knowledge, and the adaptation to cultural diversity (including policies, values, structure, and services), accounting for unique characteristics such as their socioeconomic level, level of acculturation, and experience with the service system. Cross and colleagues asserted that it was difficult for clinicians to practice in a culturally competent fashion without the support of practicing within a culturally competent organization.

The cultural sensibility model. This model conceptualized by Karnik and Dogra (2010) takes the cultural competence approach further in that it considers cultural differences across all populations. The cultural competence model arose from concerns around minority mental health disparities and the need to address those disparities within the treatment setting. The cultural sensibility model proposes that culture is an underlying factor in all human interaction, whether one is from a minority or majority population (or in the case of immigrants and refugees from the immigrant or host culture). This model advocates integrating cultural considerations in all clinical interactions and treatment approaches and including factors that go beyond race and ethnicity, such as religion and spirituality, gender, socioeconomic status, and regional cultural differences within a nation. This model is particularly useful in addressing the mental health needs of immigrants and refugees as they relocate to communities that themselves are very diverse in their composition and values even though they belong to the same host nation and culture. Additionally, this is a model that will be increasingly applicable as the United States and other Western nations become more pluralistic and diverse, with no majority ethnic, racial, or cultural population.

The community systems of care model. The cultural competence model for mental health services arose from the community systems of care model, first conceptualized by Stroul and Friedman (1986). The latter model arose out of an era in the 1970s and early 1980s when children with mental health needs were increasingly being served in out-of-home residential programs that removed them from their families and their community supports. This model advocates for mental health services to incorporate a number of different values oriented to maintain tenure and function in the home community and connection to natural supports, such as families, friendship networks, and natural institutions (e.g., schools and faith communities) while receiving effective mental health services.

The principles included in the community systems of care model are comprehensive services in the least restrictive environment, provided across service agencies in a coordinated fashion; individualized services that are tailored to the needs and strengths of the patient and family; inclusion of families as full participants in care planning and treatment (and increasingly the participation of youth as well); case management and the central coordination of such systems (including the delivery of both formal services and natural and supplementary supports); the promotion of early identification and preventive services; smooth transitions from pediatric to adult services (and, it could be added, increasingly from adult to elder services); and services that are sensitive to cultural differences and special needs (e.g., sexual and gender diversity, physical health conditions, and developmental and intellectual differences).

Although this model was initially conceptualized and applied within children's mental health services, its principles have been increasingly adopted in the design and implementation of mental health services for older populations. Service models such as assertive community treatment (ACT) programs and intensive case management (Stein & Santos, 1998) are quite consistent with the community system of care model.

Various authors have appropriately placed the delivery of mental health services to immigrant and refugee populations within such a broader systems approach for comprehensively addressing bio-psycho-social needs, with basic survival and support needs needing to be universally available, while more highly specialized mental health services are delivered in a progressively escalated and selected manner.

For example, Hodes (2002) presented a multitier model for the delivery of mental health services to refugee children, organized as follows:

Tier 1. Primary care, schools, and other community agencies; address minor behavioral difficulties

Tier 2. Child mental health professionals in schools or health centers; manage youngsters with troubling symptoms or minor disorders;

inform Tier 1 and 2 professionals and facilitate referral to Tier 3 services (e.g., outreach mental health services to schools)

Tier 3. Multidisciplinary administrative teams teams manage youngsters with severe and complex problems, with high levels of comorbidity with greater social/family impairment (can occur in schools or clinics)

Tier 4. Highly specialized out- or inpatient regional services, with only small numbers of young refugees needing psychiatric admission, but young refugees overrepresented; as likely as other adolescents to be admitted because of psychosis, deliberate self-harm, and aggressive outbursts

APPLICATION OF UNDERLYING PRINCIPLES IN THE MENTAL HEALTH CARE OF IMMIGRANTS AND REFUGEES

The principles of cultural competence and community-based systems of care were used as the basis to craft the "Practice Parameter for Cultural Competence in Child and Adolescent Psychiatric Practice" by the American Academy of Child and Adolescent Psychiatry (Pumariega et al., 2013). The practice parameter presented a structure for the implementation of these principles, supported by the available evidence at the time. It provides a useful structure within which to conceptualize important elements of mental health care for immigrant and refugee populations. Next, we outline the key recommendations made in the practice parameter that are most relevant to the care of immigrants and refugees, some with programmatic intervention examples.

Recommendation 1. *Clinicians should identify and address barriers (economic, geographic, insurance, cultural beliefs, stigma, etc.) that may prevent culturally diverse people and their families from obtaining mental health services.*

Minority populations in general, and immigrants and refugees in particular, utilize fewer mental health services than host culture mainstream populations and often may not remain engaged in such services. Multiple systemic and logistical barriers interfere with timely access to services, including financial needs, location of services and transportation, lack of adequate insurance, poorly understood bureaucratic procedures, and lack of linguistic support (Williams & Westermeyer, 1986). Though many traditional cultural values and beliefs are a source of strength and support for immigrant and refugee families, some can act as barriers to mental health services. These include cultural values that are often mobilized to deal with immediate stressors and needs, such as fatalism, spirituality, familism (leading one to keep problems within the family); cultural commitment (e.g., using only culturally sanctioned helping approaches like religious counseling and traditional healers); and help seeking expectations. These beliefs and values change over time with increasing acculturation. For example, Abe-Kim, Takeuchi, and Hwang (2002) found that rates of mental health–related service use, subjective satisfaction, and perceived helpfulness of services varied by birthplace and generation; U.S.-born Asian Americans used services at higher rates than their immigrant counterparts, and third-generation or later individuals had the highest (62.6%) rates of service use in the previous year.

Stigma is also a powerful barrier to timely access to treatment and services by refugees and immigrants (Williams & Westermeyer, 1986). In many cultures, mental illness has major negative connotations, leading to the fear of double discrimination, which prevents immigrant and refugee families from accessing services. This is especially true within communities and political climates where immigrants and refugees are perceived as and accused of posing an added burden to society. Additionally, psychiatric and mental health services and nations of origin are often oriented to severe conditions and restrictive care. These perceptions can become self-reinforcing when emergency services are needed due to the progressive aggravation of mental health and psychiatric conditions and the traumatic impact of suddenly receiving a more restrictive level of care or involuntary care. Families may mistrust mental health service agencies given their past histories of discrimination and disregard for cultural needs, as well as fear of persecution in the context of documentation difficulties and adverse political climates.

Initial psychological first aid services and outreach services in refugee camps and receiving communities, as well as mobilization of human/social support services, are important first steps in improving access and delivering basic mental health services for immigrants and refugees. Programs that address support services and offer assistance in resettlement, social and economic supports, interpreter services, and orientation to host nation society, customs, and laws are also essential components. Subsequent mental health services can be based within school or community organizations to reduce stigma and reduce barriers to access. Governmentally supported relocation programs as well as ethnic-specific programs for refugees have predominated, with the ability to provide more direct supports for affected populations (also see programmatic examples under Recommendation 11).

Recommendation 2. *Clinicians should conduct the evaluation in the language in which the child and family are proficient.*

Recommendation 3. *Clinicians should understand the impact of dual-language competence on the child's adaptation and functioning.*

Language-based communication is critical in obtaining accurate clinical information and establishing a therapeutic alliance. Many immigrants and especially refugees, however, are not fluent in English and may not be able to fully participate in the clinical process, resulting in significantly lower utilization of mental health services (Abe-Kim et al., 2007; Sentell, Shumway, & Snowden, 2007). Lack of appropriate linguistic ability or interpreter support has been associated with misdiagnosis and adverse clinical outcomes (Flores et al., 2003; Malgady & Constantino, 1998). In these cases, clinicians should either obtain linguistic support through qualified interpreters or possess demonstrable proficiency in the target language. Unfortunately, translation and interpretation are often considered menial or informal tasks in the clinical process, as reflected by the use of untrained interpreters without regard to impact on the identified patient and family members (Four Racial Ethnic Panels, 1999). Language brokering, the practice of having children act as interpreters between parents and medical and school authorities, is commonly seen among immigrant and refugee families. However, it should be avoided, particularly when the patient is the language broker. High language brokering contexts have been associated with higher levels of family stress, lower parenting effectiveness, as well as poorer mental health and academic adjustment by the use of an interpreter (Martinez, McClure, & Eddy, 2009).

Telephonic interpretation services enable 24-hour access and a wide range of available languages but are not ideal due to their inability to convey nonverbal communication. Interpreters should have proper training in the skill of interpretation, the content area being discussed, and knowledge about the population culture in question, if at all possible coming from the population. They should serve as integral members of the clinical team, serve as cultural consultants when understanding of the family's culture is needed, and interpret all of verbal and nonverbal interactions. Any educational materials and rating or diagnostic instruments should be translated to the language of the family members or child, with semantic equivalency and reliability/validity in the target language established as much as possible.

Language acquisition and dual-language competency is another critical area, particularly for immigrant and refugee children who are continuing their education and the host nation. An estimated 20% of American children 18 and under grow up exposed to two languages, which is actually below the percentage of many other polyglot nations. Learners of "English as a second language" (ESL; defined as any language learned after age 3, which is the end of the critical period for rapid language acquisition) constitute the majority of dual-language children in America. After English, the most common home language in the United States is Spanish. Grammatical and other language errors made by a child learning a second language should not be confused with language disorders. On the other hand, deficits associated with psychiatric and language disorders (e.g., auditory–verbal working memory deficits) may slow the acquisition of a second language. Specialized consultation and assessment over time by a speech/language pathologist with expertise in dual-language children may be necessary to differentiate normal from disordered language acquisition (Toppelberg & Collins, 2010).

There is evidence that maintaining the first (home) language is important in accessing family and community protective factors and other benefits. Despite this evidence, there has been a poorly substantiated practice of recommending to parents that they discontinue speaking the home language to a child who is facing language, cognitive, or other delays. Children with linguistic or other deficits may become overwhelmed by the additional cognitive and linguistic demands of dual-language learning. However, recommendations to discontinue learning the home language may have potentially serious consequences and should not be made lightly and should involve speech and language professionals. This is especially due to the adverse consequences of and ability to communicate with one's parents and extended family in the immigrant context, especially during adolescence. Additionally, supporting academic achievement in the child's primary language has been shown to support learning stability and transition to the acquired language, particularly in the context of multiple moves across schools and neighborhoods, which are often associated with immigrant and refugee status.

Recommendation 4. *Clinicians should be cognizant that cultural biases might interfere with their clinical judgment and work towards addressing these biases.*

There is much evidence of cultural and racial disparities in diagnostic assessment, treatment outcomes, and the quality of healthcare (Alegria, Vallas, & Pumariega, 2010). Stereotyping, biases, and uncertainties in healthcare providers can lead to unequal treatment (Institute of Medicine, 2002). When the patient's presentation or diagnosis is unclear, physicians may inadvertently overrely on behavioral or clinical stereotypes of specific groups at the expense of focusing on the patient's unique experience, clinical presentation, or sociocultural context. Prejudice, an unjustified negative attitude based on a person's group membership, also forms part of the stereotypes. There is considerable empirical evidence that people who are not overtly biased and do not believe they are prejudiced experience implicit and at times negative racial/ethnic attitudes and stereotypes (Cross et al., 1989).

In mental health care, a common phenomenon influenced by stereotyping and bias is that of countertransference. Countertransference can range from bias against a population or any immigrants to overidentification or "rescue fantasies" in working with these populations. It is important to avoid stereotypes or cognitive shortcuts in the clinical evaluation of immigrants and refugees (e.g., assuming that all suffer from post-traumatic stress disorder [PTSD] vs. that all are highly resilient). Mental health assessments need to be individualized and contextualized to account for baseline adaptation, socioeconomic background, dose and intensity of trauma-related stressors, availability of family and other supports versus lack of validation/rejection, genetic factors for psychopathology (though difficult to obtain histories), and other unique factors.

Recommendation 5. *Clinicians should apply knowledge of cultural differences in developmental progression, idiomatic expressions of distress, and symptomatic presentation for different disorders to the clinical formulation and diagnosis.*

Motor, language, cognitive, and social development can differ across cultures. These differences may result from developmental expectations consistent with different cultural value systems. Such differences, when viewed outside their cultural context, could lead to the misidentification of developmental regression or psychopathology (Pumariega & Joshi, 2010; Pumariega, Rothe, & Rogers, 2009). Normative expressions of psychological or emotional distress also differ across cultures. Idioms of distress are linguistic or somatic patterns of experiencing and expressing illness or general stress. Idioms of distress do not generally correspond to diagnostic categories. They can at times be alternative means of expression for psychiatric disorders as defined by Western psychiatry, such as depression or anxiety disorders. However, they can also be expressions of psychological distress unique to given cultures. More complex expressions of illness or distress are termed *cultural syndromes* (Kirmayer, 2001).

Idioms of distress and cultural syndromes can often be mistaken for more serious psychopathology, while they are often normal variants of expression of distress. For example, *ataques de nervios* (a reaction combining anxiety, agitation, and dissociation common among Latinos of Caribbean origin) can be confused with psychotic reactions, while *falling out* (a syndrome of acute paralysis and dissociation seen among populations of African origin) can be mistaken for catatonia. There also are multiple variants for the expression of depression and anxiety across cultures spanning Asia, Africa, and the Middle East. With immigrant and refugee populations, it is important to distinguish normal variants of grieving or acute stress reactions (which are common experiences) versus signs and symptoms of serious psychopathology.

The *DSM-5* (*Diagnostic and Statistical Manual of Mental Disorders, Fifth Edition*) "Outline for Cultural Formulation" provided a useful framework for assessing sociocultural aspects of the immigrant or refugee patient's mental health and relating these to the clinical formulation (Aggarwal, 2010; Lewis-Fernández, Aggarwal, Hinton, Hinton, & Kirmayer, 2016). It calls for a systematic assessment across five distinct categories: (1) *cultural identity of the individual* (including racial, ethnic, or cultural reference groups; degree of involvement with the culture of origin vs. host culture, religion, socioeconomic background, place of origin, migrant background, and sexual orientation); (2) *cultural conceptualization of illness* (including the influence of cultural beliefs on the individual's experience, conceptualization, and expression of symptoms or problems); (3) *psycho-social stressors and cultural features of vulnerability and resilience*, including key stressors and supports in the individual's sociocultural environment (e.g., religion, family, and social supports); (4) *cultural features of the relationship between the individual and the clinician* (e.g., dynamics of differences based on culture, socioeconomic, language, and social status that may cause differences in communication and influence diagnosis and treatment); and (5) *overall cultural assessment,* summarizing the implications of the aspects mentioned for diagnosis, plan of care, and other clinically relevant issues. It also includes various interviews and modules to conduct systematic assessment based on the formulation.

Recommendation 6. *Clinicians should assess the history of immigration-related losses or traumas and community trauma (violence, abuse) in the child and family and address these concerns in treatment.*

Migration results in risks and stressors unique to immigrants; any of these risks and stressors (or more likely a combination) can have significant adverse mental health consequences. These stressors can be divided into (1) premigration stress, such as exposure to violence, persecution, and torture in the country of origin; (2) migration stress, including the disruption and separation of families, traumatic journeys, detention in refugee camps, and various forms of victimization (e.g., abuse by smugglers); (3) postmigration and acculturation stress, resulting from low levels of education and job skills, living in high-risk neighborhoods, with high exposure to crime and violence and overcrowded, poor quality inner-city schools (Orfield & Yun, 1998; Sack, 1998). The stresses of immigration on the family can also result in domestic violence and criminal activity. Additionally, immigrants and their families often face unique stressors of prejudice and discrimination associated with their status, as well as those experienced by nonimmigrant minorities. As a result of these stressors, immigrants, children of immigrants, and second-generation children of immigrants are generally at increased risk for mental health problems, including anxiety, depression, substance abuse, and PTSD. Parental emotional well-being, family and community support, and supportive peer relationships can mitigate or aggravate these problems (Hovey & King, 1996; J. McFarlane, Groff, O'Brien, & Watson, 2003; Pumariega & Rothe, 2010).

Immigration to the United States can lead to complex patterns of family fragmentation and reunification. To become established, parents may immigrate before their children, leaving them with relatives in the country of origin. Children are then brought to the United States years later with hopes of reunification and giving them a better life. Children who have experienced such separations or losses have a higher risk for later developing depression, conduct, and substance abuse disorders compared to other immigrant children. Refugee and undocumented children and their families are exposed to more sudden and unpredictable separations from family and other supports, as well as uncertainty about permanency of residency (relocation vs. return to their homeland). Adolescent victims of war and genocide are at an even higher risk of conduct disorder, aggressive and sexual acting-out behaviors, substance abuse, depression, and PTSD. Those exposed to traumatic crossings and confinement in refugee camps experience silent symptoms of PTSD, which often go unnoticed by teachers and other adults. Treatment of immigrant and refugee children as well as inner-city minority children must address traumatic exposure from these various sources, use evidence-based interventions that address the impact of trauma in the child and family, and provide for significant community support for these children and their families (Pumariega & Rothe, 2010).

Recommendation 7. *Clinicians should evaluate and address the level of acculturation and presence of acculturation stress and intergenerational acculturation family conflict in immigrant and refugee children and families.*

Acculturation directly impacts the developmental task of identity, which is a lifelong developmental task but a critical one during adolescence. Peers and family members serve as "mirrors" against which the self is reflected and involved. For diverse children and youth, particularly immigrants and refugees, this mirroring comes from two sources: the traditional cultural environment of the home and the mainstream cultural environment of peers, school, and the broader community, which can often result in conflicting images. Immigrant children and youth often face significant pressures to assimilate into mainstream society through peer interaction as well as media images that communicate implicit threats of social and economic marginalization. Research supports the best adaptational outcomes of acculturation for youth are associated with the development of a *bicultural identity*, where the immigrant youth remain rooted in their culture of origin (often mediated by learning the home language) but have the necessary knowledge and interpersonal skills to successfully navigate the host culture (often resulting in a hyphenated identity) (Pumariega & Rothe, 2010; Rothe et al., 2010). However, immigrant children and families face other potential outcomes that can have adverse consequences, including *marginalization, overassimilation, cultural separation*, or *negative identification*, the last being a form of marginalization where the youth is openly hostile to both the culture of origin and the host culture and adopts values and practices antithetical to both (e.g., adoption of gang culture or even ideological extremism) (Erikson, 1968; Rothe et al., 2010).

Acculturation stress is distress and internal conflict resulting from adaptation to a new host culture, including internal cultural value conflicts and external pressures to assimilate, as well as facing racism and discrimination from the host culture. It can also result from the loss of protective aspects of the traditional culture that help with developmental stresses (e.g., religious beliefs, natural taboos) while not yet adopting counterpart beliefs from the host culture. Acculturation stress can increase the risk for psychopathology, including substance abuse, depression, anxiety, suicidality, conduct disturbance, and PTSD (Duarte et al., 2008; Rothe, et al., 2010).

It can also aggravate preexisting conditions. For example, 1 year after immigration, the rates of PTSD decreased more in Bosnian than Southeast Asian immigrant youth who were victims of ethnic cleansing. Becker, Weine, and Vojvoda (1999) speculated that fewer cultural differences between the country of origin and the host country accounted for the better adaptation of Bosnian refugees to the United States. A number of studies have found associations between a stronger ethnic identity with lower acculturative stress, better academic performance, better psychological adaptation, and fewer externalizing and internalizing symptoms, but greater awareness of discrimination. Parental stress and family separations can adversely affect acculturative stress, while positive family relations can ameliorate it (Pumariega & Rothe, 2010; Rothe et al., 2010).

Another significant source of acculturative stress within immigrant families is that of *acculturative family distancing*. This is a phenomenon that develops when more traditional parents who are reticent to adapt to the host culture encounter the behaviors, demands for greater independence, and challenges to authority from their more assimilated children, particularly adolescent children. In its more extreme forms, this process often results in significant family conflict and an increased risk for various forms of psychopathology, including substance use disorders, conduct disorders, depression, and suicidality (Hwang & Wood, 2009;Portes & Rumbaut, 1996; Szapocznik & Kurtines, 1989).

Cognitive behavioral, psychodynamic, and family therapy approaches can all be used in addressing acculturation stress and acculturative family distancing. An evidence-based family therapy model, brief strategic family therapy (Santisteban et al., 2003), originally developed with Latino immigrant families, has as its main focus addressing acculturative family distancing through the development of mutually empathic cultural understanding by parents and youth (with greater willingness by parents to acculturate and greater awareness by youth of their traditional heritage), as well as promotion of effective parenting and communication techniques.

Recommendation 8. *Clinicians should make special efforts to include family members and key members of traditional extended families, such as grandparents or other elders, in assessment, treatment planning, and treatment.*

Recommendation 9. *Support parents to develop appropriate behavioral management skills consonant with their cultural values and beliefs.*

In the collectivist cultures where most immigrants and refugees originate, people view themselves primarily as members of groups and usually consider the needs of the group over the needs of individuals. Extended family involvement may be the only acceptable model of addressing emotional and mental health problems. In contrast, in individualistic cultures, these problems are addressed by the individual or immediate relatives within the nuclear family. Therapeutic engagement of diverse families may call for strategies that involve extended family members and nonblood kin. Their involvement may be important in obtaining necessary collateral input for appropriate diagnosis, subsequent treatment recommendations, and treatment adherence (Chatters, Taylor, & Jayakody, 1994). Although clearly beneficial, this extended involvement may raise challenging issues of confidentiality. Confidentiality should be maintained in such a manner that does not interfere with communication and collaboration. During negotiation of the therapeutic alliance and contract, the providers should respect culturally established means of communication and family role functioning, but also foster family flexibility in dealing with their bicultural offspring around such issues. The use of family psychoeducation is critical for addressing questions and culturally based myths and misconceptions about psychiatric medications and forms of psychotherapy.

Clinicians should consider consulting and collaborating with traditional healers (e.g., curanderos, santeros, shamans, or religious like priests and imams), and including rituals and ceremonies in psychotherapy with patients from more traditional backgrounds. Collaboration with indigenous traditional healers can ameliorate cultural loyalty conflicts within families and also improve access to care in populations unfamiliar with or mistrusting of the medical/psychiatric model. Traditional healers are often reticent to identify themselves as collaborating with Western-trained clinicians. However, mutual respect and education in exchanging information and perspectives can foster collaboration.

An important aspect of family psychoeducation is related to childrearing and disciplinary practices. Many practices in traditional cultures at times clash with Western norms and even legal restrictions. Addressing these issues from an educational and noncritical perspective is important, while providing education and support around childrearing practices that are consonant not only with the laws of the host culture but also with the values of the culture of origin.

Recommendation 10. *Clinicians should evaluate and incorporate cultural strengths (including values, beliefs, and attitudes) in their treatment interventions to enhance the child's and family's participation in treatment and its effectiveness.*

Clinicians should assume a posture of genuine cultural curiosity in learning about the family's traditional cultural beliefs/values. A culturally competent approach (Cross et al., 1989; Sue, 2003) promotes the incorporation of beliefs, values, attitudes, and cultural rituals and practices within mental health treatment, using psychoeducational approaches to bridge traditional understanding of illness and its treatment with Western conceptualizations and its medical/scientific model. The process of participatory or shared decision-making, where cultural aspects are integrated into the implementation of evidence-based practice, is crucial to enhance culturally competent care that ensures treatment engagement (Ngo-Metzger et al., 2006). Many culturally competent psychotherapeutic approaches and interventions have been developed, including storytelling and cultural themes, symbolic rites of passage, and matching therapists according to their racial/ethnic background (Costantino, Malgady, & Rogler, 1994; Harvey & Hill, 2004; Jackson-Gilfort, Liddle, Tejeda, & Dakof, 2001).

Culturally adapted treatment modalities may have some improved effectiveness compared to standard interventions, though the evidence is mixed. Two studies using a correlational approach indicated that ethnic match between client and therapist was associated with positive outcomes following youth- and family-based treatment (Halliday-Boykins, Schoenwald, & Letourneau, 2005). A meta-analysis of 76 studies evaluating the benefit of culturally adapted mental health interventions found a moderate benefit for culturally adapted interventions (Griner & Smith, 2006). However, two smaller meta-analyses comparing culturally adapted to standard interventions did not find significant differences in effect sizes (Huey & Polo, 2008).

Recommendation 11. *Clinicians should treat culturally diverse patients and their families in familiar settings within their communities whenever possible.*

Immigrant and refugee families have difficulty navigating large mainstream healthcare institutions because of limited health literacy and knowledge of the system. They also have inherent mistrust of mainstream mental health care institutions due to cultural stigma around mental illness and negative experiences with mental health institutions in their nations of origin, which are often not only more institutional but also politically involved. As a result, immigrant and refugee families often prefer smaller ethnic-specific community clinics or clinics located within schools or ethnic neighborhoods (Akutsu, Castillo, & Snowden, 2007). School-based services are also generally well accepted and highly effective because schools are viewed as safe institutions. Clinicians should also consider home- or community-based alternatives to hospitalization due to the integral nature of community and family for emotional supports.

Any out-of-home placement should ideally be negotiated with family and patient cooperation.

The principles of treatment in the least restrictive environment are especially important given how some treatments may remove immigrants and refugees from their community, extended family, and traditional cultural supports (Pumariega et al., 2009). Involuntary hospitalization should be avoided as it tends to reexacerbate past traumas (often related to detention), contribute to new ones, and exacerbate historic mistrust of the mental system.

The principles of cultural competence (Cross et al., 1989) and community systems of care (Stroul & Friedman, 1986) promote the use of community resources and cultural strengths to facilitate effective interventions with diverse children and families. Systems of care programs have some demonstrated effectiveness in improving access to care and improving outcomes for diverse children and youth, including immigrant and refugee populations. A meta-analysis of services utilization data versus home community composition for the federal Comprehensive Children's Mental Health Initiative communities (Miech et al., 2008) found that these programs successfully reach disadvantaged and minority youth, including reducing mental health disparities and achieving equivalent clinical and functional outcomes as for mainstream culture Caucasian youth (Fisher, Sukumar, Manteuffel, & Stephens, 2005; Miech et al., 2008).

There are some notable examples of school-based mental health prevention and intervention programs tailored to the needs of immigrant and refugee youth populations that hew to the community-based services model. The AMIGO program (Rousseau & Guzder, 2008) provides mental health services to 15 elementary schools in Montgomery County, Maryland. Its goals are to enhance students' personal, social, and academic development; improve family communication and reduce stress; cope with grief and loss associated with migration; address language differences between home and school; and facilitate the cultural adjustment of recent arrivals. It provides a wide array of mental health services, including individual, group, and family therapy; in-home and crisis intervention; school consultation; interagency collaboration; and parent education/supports. It works to build trust by addressing families' basic subsistence needs and facilitating access to services through home outreach. In program evaluation responses from families and youth, AMIGO activities were perceived as bringing a significant improvement to the lives of the children and their families.

The Robert Woods Johnson Foundation funded a school-based prevention and intervention program, Caring Across Communities (McNeeley, Sprecher, & Bates, 2010); it involves 15 model sites, each working with defined immigrant and refugee populations in different U.S. communities. Its goal is to engage schools, families, students, mental health agencies, and other community organizations to build effective, easily accessed services for children and youth. One of the programs is Project SHIFA, based out of the Boston Children's Hospital Center for Refugee Trauma. Its target population is Somali refugee children and families in Boston, with the goal of provision of trauma-informed care to Somali youth that is accessible and effective. Its main intervention, Trauma Systems Therapy (TST) for Refugees, addresses emotional regulation of traumatized refugee children within the social environment and includes strong advocacy, systems integration, and community-based participation. Multiple mental health disciplines are involved in the delivery of a continuum of services, including prevention (community and teacher education), early identification/intervention (youth groups), and intensive intervention focused on individual youth and families and also the provision of support and legal services. Another program is BieneStar in Durham, North Carolina, which is a partnership between the Duke Division of Community Health, El Centro Hispano of Durham, Durham Public Schools, and the Center for Child and Family Health. Its focus is three elementary schools in Durham Public Schools with large immigrant Hispanic/Latino enrollment. Its goals are to provide bilingual culturally responsive preventive and direct mental health services integrated within schools, targeting newly arrived Latino parents and their children. BieneStar provides outreach to parents through bilingual staff, school-wide education about mental and behavioral health issues, parent and family orientation and education groups, support and legal services, and cultural competence training for teachers and other staff throughout school year.

The U.S. Department of Education, Office of English Language Acquisition (2016), has promoted the development of newcomer programs for newly arrived refugee children and families in "destination cities" where refugees are relocated. These are short-term programs (usually 6–18 months) for recent immigrant students. The goals for these programs are to address limited English proficiency, low literacy, and limited schooling; to ease transition, other services for students may include healthcare, mental health care, career counseling, and tutoring. These programs sometimes serve families, providing outreach, adult ESL, orientation to the community, and assistance accessing social services, healthcare, housing, and employment. Schools partner with the community to serve parents and families. Effective newcomer programs recognize they provide temporary, short-term supports.

After participation in newcomer programs, students will continue to require additional support to meet high academic standards in mainstream classrooms. These programs constitute a first step in a long-term process where students transition into increasingly integrated settings with decreasing levels of support. Teachers must coordinate curriculum and instruction across newcomer programs, ESL/bilingual programs, and mainstream classes (Rivera, Lesaux, Kieffer, & Rivera, 2006). Examples of newcomer model programs include the Student Intake Center of the Dallas, Texas, Independent School District, part of a multilingual enrichment program (Dallas, TX, Independent School District, 2018, https://www.dallasisd.org/) and the ESL Newcomer Academy of Jefferson County Schools, Kentucky (Jefferson County Schools, 2018, https://www.jefcoed.com/).

A more active treatment model is Cognitive Behavioral Therapy for Traumatic Stress (CBITS; Kataoka et al., 2003). It started out as the Mental Health for Immigrant Program (MHIP), implemented in the Los Angeles Independent School District but now replicated nationally. It is a school-based program delivering multilevel cognitive behavioral therapy (CBT) interventions (group, individual, psychoeducational), delivered by educators and mental health professionals using a manualized format. The model addresses acculturation stress and cultural trauma and has demonstrated significant reductions in PTSD and depressive symptoms and improvements in function.

Recommendation 12. *Clinicians should preferentially use evidence-based psychological and pharmacological interventions specific for the ethnic/racial population of the immigrant patient and family.*

The racial/ethnic disparity in the evidence base for various psychiatric and psychological interventions continues to be a result of a lack of evaluation of such interventions in culturally diverse populations and the overrepresentation of Euro-Americans in study populations. In recent years, however, there has been a growing literature evaluating the efficacy of various forms of psychotherapy and community-based interventions in diverse populations, including immigrant and refugee populations. It is incumbent on clinicians to preferentially utilize evidence-based interventions with specific population-based evidence.

Psychotherapeutic interventions with refugees require their being trauma informed or with a focus on trauma. The following interventions have been widely used or specifically address the impact of trauma in refugees (Ehntholt & Yule, 2006):

Cognitive behavioral interventions for PTSD. These interventions are based on learning and information-processing theories. Learning theory proposes that changes in behavior are thought to result from influencing antecedents and consequences. Information-processing theory proposes that cognitions drive behavior; therefore, altering cognitions can lead to changes in behavior and affect. Cognitive behavioral work generally draws on both theories through the application of behavioral techniques, as well as examination of the cognitive interpretations and attributions about events made by the person. Interventions range from problem-solving strategies to exposure methods or cognitive techniques aimed at modifying distorted thinking.

Testimonial psychotherapy. Testimonial psychotherapy was developed specifically for adult survivors of multiple traumatic events over an extended period of time, such as torture or severe human rights abuses.

This approach utilizes recording, often with the assistance of a recording device, of an individual's verbal account of what the individual has experienced. The account is then revised jointly by the individidual and therapist during subsequent sessions until it forms a coherent written narrative. The signing of the completed document signals a formal end to the process and then is presented to human rights organizations or others as evidence of an individual's experience of abuse. The document may be used for legal or political purposes. The integrative nature of this method enables an individual to assimilate fragmented traumatic memories with their accompanying affective and cognitive states, as well as within their sociopolitical and historical context. Testimonial psychotherapy also fits the oral tradition of storytelling found in many traditional cultures.

Narrative exposure therapy (NET). NET is an innovative approach that combines elements of testimonial psychotherapy with cognitive behavioral techniques. It was developed as a short-term treatment based on the principles of cognitive behavioral exposure therapy but using an adapted narrative approach for exposure. It is better suited to address the needs of victims of organized violence who have experienced multiple traumatic events and find it difficult to identify the worst event. The individual constructs a narrative about his or her whole life from birth to the present while giving a detailed report of all traumatic events. One of the goals of this approach is to reduce PTSD symptoms by confronting the individual with memories of the traumatic event. Improvement of symptoms may be due to not only habituation of emotional responses but also the reconstruction of distorted and fragmented autobiographical traumatic memories into a coherent narrative.

Eye movement desensitization and reprocessing (EMDR) uses bilateral stimulation when processing traumatic memories in individuals with PTSD. With this method, the person is often asked to conjure an image of his or her traumatic event while the therapist simultaneously moves his or her finger in front of the young person's eyes in a rhythmic, lateral motion. The treatment combines both exposure and distraction or "dual attention." Findings from available studies must be interpreted with caution due to the lack of control groups, small sample sizes, and the mixture of psychotherapeutic methods with EMDR. Improvements could be due to such factors as natural recovery over time, the granting of permanent residence, or treatment components other than EMDR. Although promising, further research is needed.

Some reviews and meta-analyses have examined the relative effectiveness and value of these and other psychotherapeutic interventions with traumatized immigrants and refugees. Crumlish and O'Rourke (2010) conducted a systematic review of randomized controlled trials of the treatment of PTSD among refugees and asylum seekers, rated trials with a risk-of-bias table, and drew conclusions about the evidence for individual therapies. Ten randomized, controlled trials (n = 528) met the search criteria. The trials were small, and allocation concealment and blinding were inadequate. No treatment was firmly supported, but there was evidence for NET and CBT.

C. McFarlane and Kaplan (2012) identified 40 studies from 1980 to 2010 that investigated interventions for adult survivors of torture and trauma. Population subtypes included resettled refugees, asylum seekers, displaced persons, and persons resident in their country of origin. Settings included specialized services for torture and trauma, specialized tertiary referral clinics, community settings, university settings, as well as psychiatric and multidisciplinary mental health services. Interventions were delivered as individual or group treatments and lasted from a single session to 19 years' duration and included culturally adapted CBT with selective serotonin reuptake inhibitors (SSRIs), NET, trauma-focused therapy, psychoeducation, group therapy, and testimonial therapy. The studies employed randomized controlled trials, nonrandomized comparison studies, and single-cohort follow-up studies. In all, 36 of the 40 studies (90%) demonstrated significant improvements on at least one outcome indicator after an intervention. Most studies (60%) included participants who had high levels of post-traumatic stress symptomatology. Improvements in symptoms of post-traumatic stress, depression, anxiety, and somatic symptoms were found following a range of interventions. Little evidence was available with regard to the effect on treatment outcomes of the amount, type, or length of treatment; the influence of patient characteristics; maintenance of treatment effects; and treatment outcomes other than psychiatric symptomatology.

Lambert and Alhassoon (2015) conducted a meta-analysis of randomized controlled trials of psychotherapeutic intervention for traumatized adult refugees. They compared 13 trauma-focused therapies to control groups from 12 studies. The aggregate effect sizes for the primary outcome, PTSD, and depression were large. They used metaregression to evaluate potential moderators of the PTSD effect size. Number of sessions significantly predicted the magnitude of the effect size, and studies that utilized an active control group (e.g., supportive counseling) had a significantly smaller effect size than those with a passive control group. There were no differences in outcome for studies where an interpreter was used versus those where no interpreter was used. There also was no difference in outcome based on type of PTSD assessment. Results provided evidence for the efficacy of trauma-focused models for treating refugees.

All of these studies concluded the need for more in-depth research into the contexts of the delivery of these interventions as well as better evaluation of the elements that contributed to their effectiveness.

Some authors, however, pointed to the limitations of psychotherapeutic interventions in addressing the needs of refugees and traumatized immigrants. Miller (1999) examined the primary role of psychotherapy and other clinic-based services in addressing the mental health needs of political refugees. He found two key factors contributing to adverse mental health outcomes for refugees: (1) the pervasiveness of psychological distress within refugee communities, coupled with the reluctance of many refugees to utilize formal psychological and psychiatric services; (2) a considerable amount of the distress reported by refugees related not to prior exposure to violent events but to a host of exile-related stressors and losses, such as loss of community and social network, changes in socioeconomic status and concerns about economic survival, loss of meaningful structure and activity in daily life, and loss of significant social roles. He concluded that, while psychotherapy can play an important adjunctive role, exile-related stressors may most effectively be addressed through targeted community and culturally based interventions.

Murray, Davidson, and Schweitzer (2010) surveyed refugee research, examined empirical evaluations of therapeutic interventions in resettlement contexts, and provided recommendations for best practices and future directions in resettlement countries. The resettlement interventions found to be most effective typically targeted culturally homogeneous client samples and demonstrated moderate-to-large outcome effects on aspects of traumatic stress and anxiety reduction. They felt that further evaluation is needed for the array of psychotherapeutic, psycho-social, pharmacological, psychoeducational, and community-based interventions utilized with these populations. They also identified a need for increased training and funding to implement longitudinal interventions that work with clients from refugee backgrounds through the stages of resettlement.

More generic psychotherapeutic interventions that have evidence for diverse populations include CBT for depression and anxiety (Huey & Polo, 2008; Pina et al., 2003; Pumariega et al., 2009); interpersonal psychotherapy for treatment of depression; group CBT for anxiety disorders in African Americans; and manualized family therapy for the treatment of substance abuse (Santisteban et al., 2003). Most of the evaluations of these interventions have involved culturally adapted protocols.

Examples of community-based interventions with racial/ethnic–specific evidence include multisystemic therapy for youth conduct disturbances, substance abuse, and suicidality (Rowland et al., 2005); CBITS (Kataoka et al., 2003); and cognitive behavioral interventions for treatment of depression (Cardemil, Reivich, Beevers, Seligman, & James, 2007). A large number of evidence-based interventions have been evaluated with minority youth with conduct problems, with over a dozen of these distinct treatments having been successfully tested in randomized trials (Huey & Polo, 2008).

Relatively less evidence exists for pharmacological interventions, but some data are available for diverse populations. For example, the Treatment of Adolescent Depression Study (TADS; Curry et al., 2006) had a 26% minority representation among its participants (principally Latino and African origin), and minority status was not found to be a significant moderator of short-term treatment outcome when using combined

CBT and pharmacotherapy. In the Multisite Treatment Study of ADHD, inner-city African Americans and Latinos required combination stimulant pharmacotherapy and cognitive behavioral intervention to achieve equal outcomes to White children, who only required stimulant pharmacotherapy (Arnold et al., 2003).

There is no specific evidence to suggest that pharmacological treatments are beneficial to young refugees with PTSD. Such treatments are usually only used as an adjunct to psychotherapeutic and psycho-social treatments for children with PTSD and are not recommended in the United Kingdom, while serotonin reuptake inhibitors, venlafaxine, and antipsychotics are recommended for adults. They should be used as a last resort if psychological therapies do not result in an improvement (National Institute for Health and Care Excellence [NICE], 2018). Clonidine has been shown to be effective for psychiatric symptoms among Cambodian refugee adults with PTSD (Kinzie & Leung, 1989). Also, studies have demonstrated some effectiveness for alpha agonists such as prazosin and clonidine for children and youth with PTSD (targeting hyperarousal and nightmares); also some limited short-term benefit was found for the use of second-generation antipsychotics and mood stabilizers for youth with severe symptoms; and a benefit from SSRIs was found for adults but not children and adolescents (Strawn, Keeshin, Del Bello, Geraciotti, & Putnam, 2010).

Recommendation 13. *Clinicians should identify ethnopharmacological factors that may influence the patient's response to medications or the patient's experience of side effects.*

There is a growing science around ethnopharmacology that has been based on the field of human molecular genetics. Although most genetic variation is shared worldwide, the relative proportion of functional genetic variants for any given gene may vary by ancestry. This in theory can lead to different racial/ethnic patterns of medication metabolism and activity and risk for side effects. The area of ethnopsychopharmacology has focused on the study of pharmacogenomic polymorphism alleles that vary in frequency across different ethnic and racial populations, raising questions about the importance of these factors in prescribing, especially with diverse immigrant populations. These include the distribution of rapid, slow, and superslow activity of cytochrome P (CYP) izoenzymes responsible for metabolizing medications in the Liver (especially CYP2D6 and CYP2D19) across different racial and ethnic populations and polymorphisms of the serotonin 2A and dopamine D_3 receptors related to antipsychotic and antidepressant treatment response and side effects, such as serotonin syndrome and extrapyramidal symptoms (Malik et al., 2010). In using such concepts concerning genetics, it is important to avoid the harmful stereotyping of the past about race and genetics and to adopt a new approach to the consideration of biological and genetic factors that serves the goals of addressing health disparities and population health.

Gene–environment interactions, such as in dietary preferences and stressful life experiences, are also important in predicting medication response and further complicate the use of race or ethnicity as a simple pharmacogenomic predictor. Such practices may change as individuals migrate to different regions and adopt the practices of their new community. For example, grapefruit juice may increase serum concentrations of nefazodone and alprazolam by affecting the CYP3A4 isoenzymes, and corn diets may increase serum concentrations of SSRIs by affecting CYP2D6 isoenzymes. Additionally, findings of interactions between stressful life events and genetic polymorphisms in serotonin transporter genes in expression of major depression may present even greater confounds for minority and immigrant populations who are acutely and chronically exposed to such stress (Kendler, Kuhn, Vittum, Prescott, & Riley, 2005; Malik et al., 2010).

It is important that clinicians inquire about and discuss the use of alternative medicinals and herbals by culturally diverse youth and families. Western medicine has not eclipsed traditional medicine, and the two are often practiced simultaneously or sequentially. Herbs and other traditional remedies sometimes have strong active ingredients, such as atropinic substances that can produce anticholinergic side effects and even toxicity. Many patients and families do not inform their doctor they are consuming these substances unless asked directly (Malik et al., 2010). When these do not pose any adverse interaction or might even be beneficial, clinician acceptance of their use can help to build the therapeutic alliance and acceptance of Western therapeutic approaches. However, one should not dismiss the potential for scientifically based effectiveness of these agents, as has been demonstrated with chamomile extract, a widely used herbal by many immigrant populations (Amsterdam et al., 2009).

Although there is great promise for pharmacogenomics to advance personalized medicine, further research is needed to identify genetic factors with definitive impact on treatment response and side effect profiles. Until such findings are available, clinicians should exercise caution in prescribing and dosing psychopharmacological agents for diverse patients. They should base decisions on the individual's clinical and familial history, migration and ancestral history, personal and familial history of pharmacological response, and dietary and natural medicinal use history (Zandi & Judy, 2010). Currently available pharmacogenomic testing may have some limited utility in cases of diverse children with mixed racial/ethnic background and atypical pharmacological response.

CONCLUSIONS

The treatment of mental health disturbance and psychiatric disorders among immigrants and refugees by its very nature needs to be highly contextualized to address the unique stressors and traumas faced by these populations, as well as be responsive to the cultural backgrounds and socioeconomic and adaptational needs inherent in the emigration and resettlement process. There can never be a "one-size-fits-all" approach, and none of the multiple factors that contribute to mental health in immigrants and refugees can be neglected or ignored.

The typical immigrant projects an aura of resilience that can be true in many respects, given all the sacrifices and travails made to reach their ultimate destinations. At the same time, communities and governments should not be misled by these external appearances, and they should be actively screening and preventing the adverse mental health consequences that can result from immigration and displacement. Unfortunately, the current political climate that promotes negativity toward immigrants and refugees contributes to shortsightedness around these issues and leads governments to ignore the evidence and the advice of experts, even when the same governments commission such work (ICE Advisory Committee on Family Residential Centers, 2016).

Because immigrants and refugees are major contributors to the growth and development of a pluralistic nation and a dynamic economy, it would be a wise investment for receiving nations to address their mental health needs, especially from the economic development perspective, aside that of the humanitarian perspective. Further research into the approaches and modalities mentioned in this chapter should also be part of that investment.

REFERENCES

Abe-Kim, J., Takeuchi, D., Hong, S., Zane, N., Sue, S., Spencer, M. S., . . . Alegria, M. (2007). Use of mental health–related services among immigrant and U.S.-born Asian Americans: Results from the National Latino and Asian American study. *American Journal of Public Health, 97*, 1–8.

Abe-Kim, J., Takeuchi, D., & Hwang, W. (2002). Predictors of help seeking for emotional distress among Chinese Americans: Family matters. *Journal of Consulting Psychology, 70*:1186–1190.

Aggarwal, N. (2010). Cultural formulations in child and adolescent psychiatry. *Journal of the American Academy of Child and Adolescent Psychiatry, 49*, 306–309.

Akutsu, P. D., Castillo, E. D., & Snowden, L. R. (2007). Differential referral patterns to ethnic-specific and mainstream mental health programs for four Asian American groups. *American Journal of Ortho-psychiatry, 77*, 95–103.

Alegria, M., Vallas, M., & Pumariega, A. (2010). Racial and ethnic disparities in pediatric mental health. *Child and Adolescent Psychiatric Clinics of North America, 19*, 759–774.

Amsterdam, J., Li, Y., Soeller, I., Rockwell, K., Mao, J., & Shults, J. (2009). A randomized, double-blind, placebo-controlled trial of oral *Matricaria recutita* (chamomile) extract therapy of generalized anxiety disorder. *Journal of Clinical Psychopharmacology, 29*(4), 378–382.

Arnold, L. E., Elliott, M., Sachs, L., Bird, H., Kraemer, H. C., Wells, K. C., . . . Wigal, T. (2003). Effects of ethnicity on treatment attendance, stimulant response-dose, and 14-month outcome in ADHD. *Journal of Consulting and Clinical Psychology, 71*:713–727.

Becker, D. F., Weine, S. M., & Vojvoda, D. (1999). PTSD symptoms in adolescent survivors of "ethnic cleansing": Results from a one-year followup study. *Journal of the American Academy of Child and Adolescent Psychiatry, 38*, 775–781.

Cardemil, E., Reivich, K., Beevers, C., Seligman, M., & James, J. (2007). The prevention of depressive symptoms in low-income minority children: Two year follow-up. *Behaviour and Research Therapy,45,*313–327.

Chatters, L. M., Taylor, R. J., & Jayakody, J. S. (1994). Fictive kinship relationships in Black extended families. *Journal of Comparative Family Studies, 25,* 297–312.

Colby, S., & Ortman, J. (2015). Projections of the size and composition of the U.S. population: 2014 to 2060. US Census Bureau, U.S. Department of Commerce; pp. 25-1143. https://www.census.gov/content/dam/Census/library/publications/2015/demo/p25-1143.pdf

Costantino, G., Malgady, R. G., & Rogler, L. H. (1994). Storytelling through pictures: Culturally sensitive psychotherapy for Hispanic children and adolescents. *Journal of Clinical Child Psychology, 23,* 13–20.

Cross, T., Bazron, B., Dennis, K., & Issacs, M. (1989). *Towards a culturally competent system of care.* Washington, DC: CASSP Technical Assistance Center, Georgetown University Child Development Center.

Crumlish, N., & O'Rourke, K. (2010). A systematic review of treatments for post-traumatic stress disorder among refugees and asylum-seekers. *The Journal of Nervous and Mental Disease, 198,* 237–251.

Curry, J., Rohe, P., Simons, A., Silva, S., Vitiello, B., Kratochvil, C., . . . TADS Team. (2006). Predictors and modifiers of acute outcome in the Treatment for Adolescents with Depression Study (TADS). *Journal of the American Academy of Child and Adolescent Psychiatry, 45,* 1427–1439.

Dallas TX Independent School District. https://www.dallasisd.org/. Accessed January 6, 2019.

Duarte, C. S., Bird, H. R., Shrout, P. E., Wu, P., Lewis-Fernández, R., Shen, S., & Canino, G. (2008). Culture and psychiatric symptoms in Puerto Rican children: Longitudinal results from one ethnic group in two contexts. *Journal of Child Psychology and Psychiatry and Allied Disciplines, 49,* 563–572.

Ehntholt, K., & Yule, W. (2006). Practitioner review: Assessment and treatment of refugee children and adolescents who have experienced war-related trauma. *Journal of Child Psychology and Psychiatry and Allied Disciplines, 47*(12), 1197–1210.

Erikson, E. H. (1968). *Identity: Youth and crisis.* New York: Norton.

Fisher, S., Sukumar, B., Manteuffel, B., & Stephens, R. (2005). A preliminary profile of Latino children and youth receiving services in systems of care communities. *Psychline,4,* 4–12.

Flores, G., Laws, M. B., Mayo, S. J., & Hardt, E. J. (2003). Errors in medical interpretation and their potential clinical consequences in pediatric encounters. *Pediatrics, 111,* 6–14.

Four Racial/Ethnic Panels. (1999). *Cultural competence standards in managed mental health care for four underserved/underrepresented racial/ethnic populations.* Rockville, MD: Center for Mental Health Services, Substance Abuse and Mental Health Administration, US Department of Health and Human Services.

Griner, D., & Smith, T. (2006). Culturally adapted mental health interventions: A meta-analytic review. *Psychotherapy (Chic), 43,* 531–548.

Halliday-Boykins, C. A., Schoenwald, S. K., & Letourneau, E. J. (2005). Caregiver-therapist ethnic similarity predicts youth outcomes from an empirically based treatment. *Journal of Consulting and Clinical Psychology, 73*, 808–818.

Harvey, A. R., & Hill, R. B. (2004). Afrocentric youth and family rites of passage program: Promoting resilience among at-risk African American youths. *Social Work, 49*, 65–74.

Hodes, M. (2002). Implications for psychiatric services of chronic civilian strife: Young refugees in the UK. *Advances in Psychiatric Treatment, 8*, 366–373.

Hovey, J., & King, C. (1996). Acculturative stress, depression, and suicidal ideation among immigrant and second-generation Latino adolescents. *Journal of the American Academy of Child and Adolescent Psychiatry, 35*, 1183–1192.

Huey, S., & Polo, A. (2008). Evidence-based psychosocial treatments for ethnic minority youth. *Journal of Clinical Child and Adolescent Psychology, 37*, 262–301.

Hwang, W., & Wood, J. (2009). Acculturative family distancing: Links with self-reported symptomatology among Asian Americans and Latinos. *Child Psychiatry and Human Development, 40*, 123–138.

ICE Advisory Committee on Family Residential Centers. (2016). *Report of the ICE Advisory Committee on Family Residential Centers.* Washington, DC: Immigration and Customs Enforcement, U.S. Department of Homeland Security. https://www.ice.gov/sites/default/files/documents/Report/2016/acfrc-report-final-102016.pdf

Institute of Medicine. (2002). *Unequal treatment: Confronting racial and ethnic disparities in health care*. Washington, DC: National Academies Press.

Jackson-Gilfort, A., Liddle, H. A., Tejeda, M. J., & Dakof, G. A. (2001). Facilitating engagement of African American male adolescents in family therapy: A cultural theme process study. *The Journal of Black Psychology, 27*, 321–340.

Jefferson County Schools. https://www.jefcoed.com/. Accessed December 16, 2018.

Karnik, N. S., & Dogra, N. (2010). The cultural sensibility model: A process-oriented approach for children and adolescents. *Child and Adolescent Psychiatric Clinics of North America, 19*(4), 719–737.

Kataoka, S., Stein, B., Jaycox, L., Wong, M., Escudero, P., Tu, W., . . . Fink, A. (2003). A school-based mental health program for traumatized Latino immigrant children. *Journal of the American Academy of Child and Adolescent Psychiatry, 42*(3), 311–318.

Kendler, K., Kuhn, J., Vittum, J., Prescott, C., & Riley, B. (2005). The interaction of stressful life events and a serotonin transporter polymorphism in the prediction of episodes of major depression: A replication. *Archives of General Psychiatry, 62*, 529–535.

Kinzie, J. D., & Leung, P. (1989). Clonidine in Cambodian patients with posttraumatic stress disorder. *The Journal of Nervous and Mental Disease, 177*, 546–550.

Kirmayer, L. (2001). Cultural variations in the clinical presentation of depression and anxiety: Implications for diagnosis and treatment. *Clinical Psychiatry, 62*(Suppl. 13), 22–28.

Lambert, J., & Alhassoon, O. (2015). Trauma-focused therapy for refugees: Meta-analytic findings. *Journal of Counseling Psychology, 62*(1), 28–37.

Lewis-Fernández, R., Aggarwal, N., Hinton, L., Hinton, D., & Kirmayer, L. (2016). *DSM-5® handbook on the cultural formulation interview*. Washington, DC: American Psychiatric Press.

Malgady, R., & Constantino, G. (1998). Symptom severity in bilingual Hispanics as a function of clinician ethnicity and language of interview. *Psychological Assessment, 10*, 120–127.

Malik, M., Lawson, W., Lake, J., & Joshi, S. (2010). Culturally adapted pharmacotherapy and the integrated formulation. *Child and Adolescent Psychiatric Clinics of North America, 19*, 791–814.

Martinez, C., McClure, H., & Eddy, J. (2009). Language brokering contexts and behavioral and emotional adjustment among Latino parents and adolescents. *The Journal of Early Adolescence,29*, 71–98.

McFarlane, C., & Kaplan, I. (2012). Evidence-based psychological interventions for adult survivors of torture and trauma: A 30-year review. *Transcultural Psychiatry, 49*(3–4), 539–567.

McFarlane, J., Groff, J., O'Brien, J., &Watson, K. (2003). Behaviors of children who are exposed and not exposed to intimate partner violence: An analysis of 330 Black, White and Hispanic children. *Pediatrics, 112*, 202–207.

McNeely, C., Sprecher, K., & Bates, D. (2010, May 24). *Comparative case study of caring across communities: Identifying essential components of comprehensive school-linked mental health services for refugee and immigrant children.* Robert Woods Johnson Foundation and Center for the Study of Youth and Political Violence and Department of Public Health University of Tennessee, Knoxville. http://healthinschools.org/wp-content/uploads/2016/10/CACFinalEvalreport.pdf. Accessed December 16, 2018.

Miech, R., Azur, M., Dusablon, T., Jowers, K., Goldstein, A. B., Stuart, E. A., . . . Leaf, P. J. (2008). The potential to reduce mental health disparities through the comprehensive community mental health services for children and their families program. *The Journal of Behavioral Health Services & Research, 35*, 253–264.

Miller, K. (1999). Rethinking a familiar model: Psychotherapy and the mental health of refugees. *Journal of Contemporary Psychotherapy, 29*(4), 283–306.

Murray, K., Davidson, G., & Schweitzer, R. (2010). Review of refugee mental health interventions following resettlement: Best practices and recommendations. *American Journal of Orthopsychiatry, 80*(4), 576–585.

National Institute for Health and Care Excellence (NICE). (2018, December). Post-traumatic stress disorder (ICE guideline [NG116]). https://www.nice.org.uk/guidance/ng116/chapter/Recommendations#management-of-ptsd-in-children-young-people-and-adults. Accessed January 6, 2019.

Ngo-Metzger, Q., Telfair, J., Sorkin, D. H., Telfair, J., Weidmer, B., Weech-Maldonado, R., & Hurtado, M. (2006). *Cultural competency and quality of care: Obtaining the patient's perspective* (Publication 963). New York: Commonwealth Fund;7–9. https://scholar.google.com/scholar_lookup?title=Cultural+Competency+and+Quality+of+Care:+Obtaining+the+Patient%E2%80%99s+Perspective&author=Q+Ngo-Metzger&author=J+Telfair&author=D+Sorkin&author=B+Weidmer&author=R+Weech-Maldonado&publication_year=2006&. Accessed January 6, 2019.

Orfield, G., & Yun, J. (1998). *Resegregation in American schools.* Cambridge, MA: Civil Rights Project, Harvard University.

Pina, A., Wendy, M., Silverman, K., Fuentes, R., Kurtines, W., & Weems, C. (2003). Exposure-based cognitive-behavioral treatment for phobic and anxiety disorders: Treatment effects and maintenance for Hispanic/Latino relative to European-American youths. *Journal of the American Academy of Child and Adolescent Psychiatry, 42,* 1179–1187.

Portes, A., & Rumbaut, R. (1996). *Immigrant America: A portrait.* Berkley: University of California Press.

Pumariega, A. J., & Joshi, S. (2010). Culture and development. *Child and Adolescent Psychiatric Clinics of North America, 49,* 661–680.

Pumariega, A. J., & Rothe, E. M. (2010). Leaving no children or families outside: The challenges of immigration. *American Journal of Orthopsychiatry, 80,* 506–516.

Pumariega, A. J., Rothe, E., Mian, A., Carlisle, L., Toppelberg, C., Harris, T., . . . the Committee on Quality Issues. (2013). Practice parameter for cultural competence in child and adolescent psychiatric practice. *Journal of the American Academy of Child and Adolescent Psychiatry, 52*(10), 1101–1115.

Pumariega, A. J., Rothe, E., & Rogers, K. (2009). Cultural competence in child psychiatric practice. *Journal of the American Academy of Child and Adolescent Psychiatry, 48,* 362–366.

Rivera, F., Lesaux, N., Kieffer, M., & Rivera, H. (2006). *Practical guidelines for the education of English language learners: Research-based recommendations for serving adolescent newcomers.* Houston, TX: Texas Institute for Measurement, Evaluation, and Statistics, the University of Houston.

Rothe, E. M., & Tzuang, D., & Pumariega, A. J. (2010). Acculturation, development and adaptation. *Child and Adolescent Psychiatric Clinics of North America, 19,* 681–696.

Rousseau, C., & Guzder, J. (2008). School-based prevention programs for refugee children. *Child and Adolescent Clinics of North America, 17,* 533–549.

Rowland, M. D., Halliday-Boykins, C. A., Henggeler, S. W., Cunningham, P. B., Lee, T. G., Kruesi, M. J. P., & Shapiro, S. B. (2005). A randomized trial of multisystemic therapy with Hawaii's Felix Class youths. *Journal of Emotional and Behavioral Disorders, 13,* 13–23.

Sack, W. (1998). Multiple forms of stress in refugee and immigrant children. *Child and Adolescent Psychiatric Clinics of North America, 7,* 153–167.

Santisteban, D. A., Perez-Vidal, A., Coatsworth, J. D., Curtines, W. M., Schwartz, S. J., LaPerriere, A., & Szapocznik, J. (2003). Efficacy of brief strategic family therapy in modifying Hispanic adolescent behavior problems and substance use. *Journal of Family Psychology, 17,* 121–133.

Sentell, T., Shumway, M., & Snowden, L. (2007). Access to mental health treatment by English language proficiency and race/ethnicity. *Journal of General Internal Medicine, 22,* 289–293.

Stein, L., & Santos, A. (1998). *Assertive community treatment of persons with severe mental illness.* New York: Norton Professional Books.

Strawn, J., Keeshin, B., Del Bello, M., Geraciotti, T., & Putnam, F. (2010). Treatment of posttraumatic stress disorder in children and adolescents: A review. *Journal of Clinical Psychiatry, 71*(7), 932–941.

Stroul, B., & Friedman, R. (1986). *A system of care for children and youth with severe emotional disturbances* (Rev. ed.). Washington, DC: Georgetown University Child Development Center, National Technical Assistance Center for Children's Mental Health.

Sue, S. (2003). In defense of cultural competency in psychotherapy and treatment. *The American Psychologist, 58*, 964–970.

Szapocznik, J., & Kurtines, W. (1989). *Breakthroughs in family therapy with drug abusing and problem youth*. New York: Springer.

Toppelberg, C., & Collins, B. (2010). Language, culture and adaptation in immigrant children. *Child and Adolescent Psychiatric Clinics of North America, 19*, 697–717.

U.S. Department of Education, Office of English Language Acquisition. (2016). *Newcomer tool kit*. Washington, DC: Author. https://www2.ed.gov/about/offices/list/oela/newcomers-toolkit/ncomertoolkit.pdf. Accessed December 16, 2018.

Williams, C., & Westermeyer, J. (Eds.). (1986). *Refugee mental health in resettlement countries.* Washington, DC: Hemisphere.

Zandi, P. P., & Judy, J. T. (2010). The promise and reality of pharmacogenetics in psychiatry. *Clinics in Laboratory Medicine, 30*, 931–974.

11

Culture, Identity, and Mental Health

Conclusions and Future Directions

Migration has been an important human activity throughout the course of history. The number of immigrants in the United States is higher than at any time in American history, but the immigrant share of the population was actually higher 90 years ago, when a large wave of immigrants arrived from Europe. There has been much recent controversy about the entry of undocumented immigrants into the United States, and this debate has contributed to an increasing anti-immigrant sentiment in a nation that paradoxically has been built by immigrants.

The 20 million second-generation Americans, adult U.S.-born children of immigrants, are substantially better off than immigrants themselves on key measures of socioeconomic attainment, identify more with the Democratic Party than with the Republican Party, and characterize themselves as liberal as opposed to conservative. This has become an important influence in the changing political demographic map in the United States.

THE IMPORTANCE OF IDENTITY AND CULTURE

Culture has been defined as a socially transmitted system of ideas that shapes behavior; categorizes perceptions; gives names to selected aspects of experience; is widely shared by members of a particular society or social group; functions as an orientational framework to coordinate and sanction behavior; and conveys values across the generations. However, the concept of culture implies that it is stationary and unchanging, so it is more accurate to refer to a people's *cultural process*, which defines the fluid and ever-changing characteristics of a culture that responds to changes in the historical and cultural contexts in which cultures are embedded (Hughes, 1993). Cultural influences are now widely recognized as having a major impact on psychological, emotional, and even cognitive development and are understood as having evolved as an adaptive mechanism in humans, allowing them to overcome challenges in more diverse environments and circumstances more rapidly than natural biologic evolution would have allowed.

Cultural differences among groups have been noted by researchers around issues such as (1) the child's developmental milestones; (2) attachment, including attachment to a particular parent, to other caretakers, or to transitional objects; (3) maternal responsiveness; (4) children's play; (5) children's emotional reactions and expression; (6) learning and preparing for social/occupational roles; and (7) the development of a particular cultural identity (Pumariega & Joshi, 2010). Cross-cultural research is also emerging in the areas of (1) theory of mind, (2) neural mapping, (3) object representation, and (4) emotional reactivity. The new neuroimaging technologies have revealed exciting discoveries in *cultural mapping* of brain functioning using functional magnetic resonance imaging (fMRI) (Chiao et al., 2009; Zhu, Zhang, Fan, & Han, 2007). These findings illustrate the dynamic influence of culture on neural representations, and that bicultural adaptation is cognitively based and neurally represented (Pumariega & Joshi, 2010).

Some of these surprising findings include an exploration into the understanding of *prejudice* associated with stereotypes, which are beliefs and categories established in children's minds in early childhood before they are taught to critically evaluate perceptions (Devine, 1989), and that some of these biases may appear as early as 3 months old, making children highly susceptible to implicit stereotypical prejudices and rejection of the "other" (Bar-Haim, Ziv, Lamy, & Hodes, 2006). Identity formation, one of the principal tasks of the passage of adolescence into adulthood, is composed of individual and social components and is closely related to the culture. A more modern definition of *identity* regards it as "the organization of self-understandings that define one's place in the world" and the synthesis of personal, social, and cultural self-conceptions, consisting of (1) personal identity, (2) social identity, and (3) cultural identity (Schwartz, Montgomery, & Briones, 2006, p. 5).

These concepts are of great value in understanding the challenges faced by immigrant adolescents, especially if they are multiracial or multiethnic, in their adaptation to the new host culture. In addition, in the area of positive adaption and psychological well-being in immigrant adolescents, new research seems to indicate that, when analyzing the interactions between *personal identity* and *cultural identity*, personal identity outweighs the latter because it is more important to understand "who one is and where one is going" than where one fits within one's ethnic group (Schwartz et al., 2006; Schwartz, Zamboanga, Weisskirch, & Wang, 2009).

SEPARATIONS AND MOURNING AS AN IMPORTANT PART OF THE IMMIGRANT EXPERIENCE

Immigrants mourn the separation from their loved ones, their parents, siblings, and sometimes their own children. They also mourn the loss of their friends and their broader network of relationships. They mourn *a sense of place and belonging* and the familiarity with the objects of everyday life, of a particular climate and geography, and departure or distancing from the early life experiences that have so much shaped their personalities. One of the major problems immigrants sometimes face is the difficulty finding their place in the new land, recovering their previous social position and the professional status they held in their native country.

Understanding the losses that the immigrant undergoes in the process of migration is fundamental to be able to design appropriate psychodynamic interventions to treat immigrants, which include (1) validating feelings of dislocation and facilitating mourning, (2) following a developmental perspective because in addition to doing the work of mourning and adaptation, the patient is *moving ahead* in his or her psycho-social development. Part of the therapist's role is to help the patient find new words to define these new experiences and the new surrounding reality, offering hope and encouragement, and acknowledging the patient's progressive accomplishments and increasing mastery over the new surroundings and new life.

IMMIGRATION-RELATED SEPARATIONS

Immigration sometimes destabilizes the family, leading to a series of family fragmentations and reunifications. In the United States, families from developing countries tend to migrate in a stepwise fashion, with parents usually arriving first, leaving the children in the temporary care of relatives back home, which is known as *child fostering*. The problems that result from these separations and reunifications often lead to psychological problems that therapists should become familiar with in order to provide the appropriate psychological care to these immigrant families.

UNDERSTANDING ACCULTURATION

Another relevant concept to keep in mind when treating immigrant populations is that of *acculturation*, which refers to the process that occurs when groups of individuals of different cultures come into continuous first-hand contact, changing the original culture patterns of either or both groups. Acculturation is even more relevant today as a result of the phenomenon of *globalization,* which defines the sociocultural climate of the twenty-first century. Globalization occurs when there is an acceleration of movement of people, products, and ideas between nations. It is characterized by an increase in fluidity between the financial and political borders between countries, which in turn increases the complexity of the everyday problems that are faced by the inhabitants of the countries (Coatsworth, 2004). The acculturation process causes change not only in the immigrant but also in the receiving culture, leading to a process of *interculturation.*

Acculturation stress is the adverse effect of psychological conflicts that result from the process of acculturation, apart from the physical health and lifestyle effects of acculturation (Berry, 1997). Some of these findings reveal that (1) first-generation immigrants are naturally selected to be a more resilient group given their decision to emigrate against many odds, with the second generation being "softer" and less resilient. (2) First-generation immigrants suppress their mental health needs in order to subsume them below their more basic and immediate needs for personal and material economic security. Once the second-generation immigrants are more comfortably established, they can then pay attention to pent-up mental health needs. (3) The second-generation immigrants may identify more readily with the devalued and denigrated concepts of their ethnic identity, adopted from the xenophobic attitudes of the host culture, which may lead to *ethnic self-hate* and higher risk for psychopathology (Escobar & Vega, 2000). (4) Family support may be strained for generation 1.5 and second-generation youth because of *acculturative family distancing* (AFD), responsible in part for the higher risk of psychopathology among immigrant youth and children of immigrants. However, most important is to keep in mind that the adult immigrant of today will someday become the American of tomorrow, and that the children of today's immigrants are a generation that should be equipped not only to understand their parents' immigrant past, but also to successfully navigate their own American futures.

TRANSNATIONAL IDENTITIES, PILGRIMAGES, AND RETURN MIGRATIONS

The concept of *transnationalism* refers to multiple interactions that link people and institutions across national borders, which has increased exponentially in the twenty-first century due to improved communication technologies and the easy and affordable access to international transportation. In addition to the country to which they have immigrated, many immigrants remain active in their countries of origin, transforming the politics, the economy, and cultural norms, such as gender relations and other aspects of everyday life. They send remittances back home and create three distinct categories of experience: (1) those who migrate, (2) those who stay behind and receive financial support from the relatives who migrated, and (3) those who do not migrate and have no sources of outside support. Remittances not only are monetary, but also include *social remittances*, which involve the exchange of ideas about democracy, gender equality, health, and community organization that deeply impact the immigrant's country of origin. Children of transnational immigrants also contribute to the process of *interculturation* in the schools they attend. Students who are native born and those who are the children of immigrants exchange ideas in which both groups acquire a better understanding and greater appreciation of diverse languages, customs, and beliefs.

Return migration is defined as the movement of emigrants back to their homelands to resettle. Various reasons are given for returning:

1. The person achieved the objective he or she had set for him- or herself.
2. The person wished to stay but was forced to return due to external factors.
3. New opportunities appeared in the person's home country that were favorable to the skills and experiences acquired abroad.
4. There are those who intended to stay but were unable to adjust due to cultural issues or homesickness.

A *pilgrimage*, in its more traditional form, is a journey to a distant place that is sacred and venerable for some reason, with the journey undertaken for devotional purposes. The personal pilgrimage in its modern secular form represents a pattern of action that can serve as an organizer to provide new integration and mastery over internal conflicts and to promote psychological growth. Sometimes, pilgrims travel to the sites not of their own childhoods, but of their family backgrounds or of their idealized cultural origins. In the case of immigrants or their descendants, pilgrimages are particularly valuable in mastering conscious and unconscious identifications with members of the previous generations. The immigrant, or descendant of an immigrant, struggles to integrate previously unmastered identifications in order to establish a personal identity as an individual while attempting to master and integrate a cultural identity that has been passed down by the previous generations of his or her family and to make the continuity from one generation to another more conflict free (Poland, 1977).

UNDERSTANDING AND TREATING REFUGEES AND SPECIAL POPULATIONS

Refugees are people who have been forced to leave their homelands due to persecution, war, or natural disasters and who face a threat to their individual safety or the safety of their family or community and who seek asylum in other countries. Those who are victims of calamities are also called refugees, but the term is more commonly used to refer to those who cross borders due to *a well-founded fear of persecution* and are *forcibly displaced*. In addition to those who do find a way to cross into other lands, there are many who cannot exit from their countries and are known as *internally displaced persons* (IDPs).

Refugees, especially children and adolescents, may demonstrate great resiliency in the face of adversity, but most refugees are exposed to multiple traumatic events that may render them vulnerable to develop mental health issues. It is very likely that the number of refugees worldwide will continue to increase as a result of regional warfare and conflict, so it is reasonable to expect continued large numbers of refugees will continue to immigrate to the United States and other developed nations to seek safety, security, and freedom (United Nations High Commissioner for Refugees [UNHCR], 2016).

Refugees have historically been a significant proportion of the immigrant population in the United States. In addition to meeting the mental health needs of refugees who arrive in the United States, our nation should develop and implement resettlement policies and practices (in human services and education) that facilitate refugees learning their new host culture while retaining the strength-based, adaptive aspects of their cultures of origin. The media and all institutions in civil society, including schools, churches, and volunteer organizations, should be recruited toward this important endeavor.

CRIMINALITY AMONG IMMIGRANTS TO THE UNITED STATES

Concerns about criminality of the foreign born were in the public debate in the United States as early as 1882, when large numbers of immigrants, predominantly from eastern Europe, began arriving on American shores. The demonization and racialization of immigrants have historically been central elements of the rhetoric surrounding U.S. immigration policy. Undocumented immigrants are portrayed as especially dangerous, sneaking into the country, committing crimes, and stealing jobs from the native born (Sohoni, 2006). Yet, despite evidence to the contrary, public opinion surveys suggest that a large number of Americans believe that continued immigration will lead to higher levels of crime, and this is particularly true when surveys emphasize the illegal status of immigrants (Adelman, Reid, Markle, Weiss, & Jaret, 2017; Ousey & Kubrin, 2009, 2018; Passel & Cohn, 2009; Sohoni & Sohoni, 2014).

Ironically, a number of studies have continued to demonstrate that immigration serves a protective function, decreasing crime rates, and that the overall crime rates are lower among immigrants than among the native born (Zatz & Smith, 2012). Studying the rates of criminality among immigrants remains a controversial issue because the data collection across the different parts of the United States is often fragmented and incomplete and because the genesis of crime involves many variables. In addition, research design varies considerably among studies (Adelman et al., 2017; Cammarota & Vaughan, 2009; Ousey & Kubrin, 2018). More research is needed in order to address many unanswered questions, such as the contribution of post-traumatic stress disorder, poverty, social marginalization, and crime among immigrants.

IMMIGRATION AND RACE

The United States was once a country with a large White majority population and a small Black minority with impenetrable color lines, but over the past four decades, immigration has increased the racial and ethnic diversity in the United States. Along with increased immigration are increases in the rates of ethnic–racial intermarriage, which is transforming the American landscape into one with a growing multiracial population. In the beginning of the twentieth century, intermarriage between Whites and other groups was very rare, but today Whites intermarry at such high rates that only one in five Whites has a spouse with an identical racial–ethnic background (Alba, 1990; Waters, 1990).

The differential rates of intermarriage suggest that racial–ethnic boundaries are more prominent for some groups than for others, for example: (1) The multiracial population seems likely to continue to grow in the foreseeable future because of increasing intermarriage. (2) Multiracial identification is not uncommon among the members of new immigrant groups, such as Asians and Latinos, particularly for those under the age of 18. (3) Multiracial identification remains relatively uncommon among Blacks compared with Asians and Latinos. (4) These patterns suggest that multiracial reporting is more likely in areas with greater levels of racial–ethnic diversity, largely brought about by the post-1965 waves of immigrants, particularly Latinos and Asians. (5) The increases in intermarriage and the growth of the multiracial population reflect a blending of races and the fading of color lines and perhaps a reduction in social distance and racial prejudice. These patterns appear to offer an optimistic portrait of weakening racial boundaries. (6) Yet, the continuing Black–non-Black divide could be a disastrous outcome for many African Americans (Lee & Bean, 2004).

It is the responsibility of the therapist to learn more about issues of race and ethnicity. It is also important for the therapist to learn about the important sociopolitical events that have occurred in American history, as well as about issues such as acculturation and identity development.

AMERICAN NARRATIVES AND IMMIGRANT NARRATIVES

People typically use stories to describe how the world works and why and how human beings do what they do. The *life story model* suggests that narrative is also a means of identity development, and that individuals construct their lives as evolving stories that support a coherent sense of self and affirm life's meaning and purpose (McAdams, 2001). In psychodynamic- and psychoanalytic-oriented therapies, the construction of narrative in the clinical encounter is now becoming recognized as an important therapeutic tool (Spence, 1982). The life story shapes and influences the identity of the narrator, but stories are also collaborative endeavors, coconstructed in the real or imagined act of being told, so the listener and the culture where the story is being told have a strong influence in shaping the story; these influences have been well documented.

It is now recognized that the psychologically healthy individual is one who is capable of holding a *coherent, dynamic*, and *meaningful narrative of the self.* Traumas tend to disrupt the narrative, so the exercise of retelling a person's life story, such as in the case of psychotherapy, can be considered as a form of *life story repair.* The creation of a narrative can also serve as a vehicle of communication that can (1) enhance a feeling of communion with others; (2) enhance a sense of agency and self-efficacy; and (3) help the person redefine his or her ultimate life concerns, such as ethical, moral, spiritual, and religious goals and values (Stein & Tuval-Mashiash, 2014).

Literary fiction with young adult immigrant protagonists is an important vehicle for understanding the realities of these new generations of Americans. Narratives are important to all human beings, but particularly in the case of immigrants, the creation of narratives gives shape to events and allows for the integration and understanding of previously challenging and troubling experiences. It creates a *new paradigm shift* where (1) the world is seen from a new perspective, (2) new options appear, and (3) new actions become possible.

TREATMENT OF IMMIGRANTS AND THE CHILDREN OF IMMIGRANTS

There is a growing demand for the provision of appropriate and effective mental health services for immigrants and refugees, now representing a larger segment of the overall population. At the same time, the process of evaluating and treating culturally diverse immigrants and their families can be complex and requires unique approaches, most of these related to the diversity in cultures and cultural values as well as the unique stressful experiences these populations have undergone. *Cultural competence* is a set of congruent behaviors, attitudes, and policies found in systems, agencies, or individual professionals that enable them to work effectively in a context of cultural difference (Cross, Bazron, Dennis, & Issac, 1989). These can be conceptualized into the cultural sensibility model and the community systems of care model.

The *cultural sensibility model* takes the cultural competence approach further in that it considers cultural differences across all populations. This model arose from concerns around minority mental health disparities and the need to address those disparities within the treatment setting. It proposes that culture is an underlying factor in all human interaction, whether one is from a minority or majority population, and advocates for integrating cultural considerations in all clinical interactions and treatment approaches, including factors that go beyond race and ethnicity, such as religion and spirituality, gender, socioeconomic status, and regional cultural differences within a nation.

The *community systems of care model* advocates for mental health services to incorporate a number of different values oriented to maintain tenure and function in the home community and connection to natural supports, such as families, friendship networks, and natural institutions (e.g., schools and faith communities) while receiving effective mental health services. The "Practice Parameter on Child and Adolescent Psychiatric Culturally Competent Care" by the American Academy of Child and Adolescent Psychiatry presented a structure for the implementation of the principles mentioned and supported by the available evidence at the time (Pumariega et al., 2013).

Research has demonstrated that immigrants and refugees underutilize mental health services, but obtain support from a series of informal community and social support organizations, such as churches (Derr, 2016). In order to effectively address the mental health disparities of this population, it is important to understand the unique service use experiences of immigrants. Future research and treatment interventions should focus on understanding and addressing the heterogeneity of the immigrant population and the gaps that currently exist in mental health service use. Finally, efforts should be made to integrate formal and informal service sectors in order to increase the outreach and treatment effectiveness to this population.

ALTERNATIVE FUTURES FOR CULTURAL IDENTITY

An Intercultural Future

A future can be envisioned where the global dissemination of cultural norms, values, and beliefs across national borders or traditional regions facilitates individuals adopting multiple ethnic/cultural identifications in a process we can term *interculturation*. As with acculturation (Rothe, Pumariega, & Sabagh, 2011), individuals can adopt aspects of different cultures and different identifications that facilitate adaptation to their ethnocultural environments. Factors such as ready and rapid travel, international business, international higher education, cross-national migration, and the global reach of media and artistic expressions can increasingly contribute to this outcome.

So far, these rapid changes in the world we live in have been conceptualized as *globalization*, though it has primarily involved Westernization of non-Western regions. However, in recent times there has also been more cross-cultural exchange with the ascendancy of various non-Western cultures, including Asian cultures, Latin American cultures, Middle Eastern cultures, and even African cultures. In fact, many youth in Western nations are increasingly fascinated by non-European or non-Western popular cultures and art forms and are adopting them into their own repertoires.

Adolescents and young adults are at the forefront of such multicultural identity formation. They are often at the leading edge of popular culture, as well as developmentally at the stage of "trying on" different identities and expressions (Erikson, 1968; Pumariega & Joshi, 2010). Youth have the freedom for such experimentation and cognitive flexibility to accommodate multiple identities, including those beyond their native cultural heritage. As with modern conceptualizations of identity, modern youth see cultural identity in a fluid manner.

Many second-generation youth with hyphenated identities due to immigration, or to the growing number of interracial and interethnic marriages across races and cultures, also contribute to an atmosphere that supports and facilitates such blended identity formation. For example, many Caucasian American youth (as well as other immigrant youth from diverse cultures around the globe) have adopted the music, dress, idioms, and mannerisms of *hip-hop* culture, which originated among inner-city African American youth to define their culture and set it apart from the culture of American mainstream youth (Rodriguez, 2006). This is much to the dismay of some African Americans, who feel that their art forms and culture are being appropriated by others in the dominant culture, though such appropriation could also be viewed as a genuine form of admiration and identification, such as in the two case examples that follow.

Case I

> A 17-year-old Caucasian American female has a mother who is involved in international business and has many dealings with Japanese companies and business people. Due in part to her negative perceptions of her very traditional American father and cliquish peers, she has long fantasied living in Japan and adopting Japanese culture. She views Japanese culture as much more nuanced than American culture and more restrained in its emotional expressions, which gives her a sense of safety and security. She has become a fan of Japanese *manga* (pictorial cartoon novels) and of Japanese popular music and performers. She is finishing high school in her hometown but is actively making plans to attend school in Japan and ultimately settle and marry there "to a nice, well-behaved Japanese guy."

Case II

> A 21-year-old second-generation Iranian American young adult male who lives with his traditional immigrant family, who themselves have assimilated to American culture after going back and forth to Iran, told his therapist that he wished he was Latino. He explained that his peers initially mistook him for Latino because of his looks, and his family did not want him to be too open about being Iranian after the 9/11 attacks in the United States. After such misidentification by others, he became curious about various Latino cultures and began to learn Spanish and develop a taste for Latin music, and he eventually wanted to move to another state that had a large Latino community so that, "I can marry a nice Mexican girl with a large, warm, and loving family."

This phenomenon has the potential to cross borders and have major social impact, culturally blurring national boundaries (this is already being seen in some instances, such as the territory between Mexico and the United States along the Southern border). This blending of cultures should help to strengthen relations between adjoining and even distant nations, promoting greater mutual understanding and cross identification (not surprisingly, many of the ambassadors representing major nations have studied or spent time in the nation where they are serving).

This multicultural identification creates significant political and economic exchange and integration, which help to slowly overcome national separation and homogeneity. For individuals living within these nations, such multicultural identifications can enhance communication and social skills as well as lead them to become more adaptable in a rapidly changing global environment.

Interculturation also has a tendency to increase egalitarianism and reduce hierarchies, or at least make them based more on merit than group membership. *Hybridization* is a similar process that takes place in the plant and animal worlds, and, as Darwin (1859) and many other scientists since have pointed out, especially geneticists, this process creates healthier and more adaptable species, so the same would appear for interculturation and psychological well-being.

A TRIBALISTIC FUTURE

The human child is expected to progress across the different stages of development toward adulthood but has the risk of engaging in regression when unable to overcome the next developmental challenge. In a similar fashion, humankind faces similar risks. One of these risks is that the process of interculturation could lead to a cultural and socioeconomic backlash that could result in growing division and global tribalism. There is already a visible trend in some nations around the world to retreat to traditional cultural values and beliefs out of fear that those cultures and their adherents will become extinct or will be overwhelmed by growing groups of "others" in their midst. Such tribalism is often fueled by xenophobia, which has been identified as a vestigial version of the primitive social hierarchies, the so-called pecking order, an ethological phenomenon seen in most avian and mammalian species where dominance and submissiveness within a species is determined to maintain order and homeostasis in the group (American Psychiatric Association, 2010). The fear of traditional privileges and economic loss by the dominant members of the group play a role in such reactions.

Currently, a fear of technology and of modernity also plays a significant role given the rapid pace of technological change and complexity. Political rhetoric can fuel the divisions that lead to tribalism, presenting intercultural exchange and globalization as a scenario of *winners and losers.* This has already occurred in many nations and cultures under despotic regimes, often with disastrous consequences, such as in Nazi Germany, the Cultural Revolution in China, the Cambodian Pol Pot regime, and others. In such contexts, cultural identity is concrete and immobile, as opposed to fluid, with little room for cultural experimentation or expression of individual differences. This greatly reduces the adaptive capacity of individuals and societies; it leads to social and economic stagnation and often results in the ultimate demise of the society that was feared in the first place.

CONCLUSIONS

Almost 13% of the American population is foreign born, and if the children of the foreign born are included, about 1 in 4 Americans can be counted as part of the recent immigrant community. Although there is lingering prejudice and popular fears of immigrants, there is growing evidence that, on balance, immigrants make a positive contribution to the American economy and society and little evidence that immigrants have an adverse impact on the wages and employment of native-born Americans (Hirschman, 2014). Moreover, immigrants and their children are disproportionately represented in a broad variety of scientific and cultural fields.

Despite the current public perceptions, an accounting of the federal fiscal system shows that immigrants (and their descendants) contribute more in taxes than they receive in benefits (Smith & Edmonston, 1997, Chapter 7). In terms of education, immigrants present an inverted bell-shaped curve and are overrepresented both among college graduates and among those with less than 12 years of schooling relative to native-born Americans (Portes & Rumbaut, 2006, Chapter 4).

Absorbing large numbers of newcomers has costs as well as benefits. The costs are immediately apparent, but some of the benefits take longer to appear, and most of the costs of these adjustments are paid by immigrants and their families. Immigrants have given up the familiarity of home in their quest for more rewarding careers and greater opportunities for their children and must also contend with a receiving society that is ambivalent, and sometimes hostile, to their presence. Immigrant parents often have to work in menial jobs, in multiple jobs, and in occupations well below the status they would have earned if they had remained in the home country. These sacrifices have meaning because immigrant parents believe that their children will have better educational and occupational opportunities in the United States than in their homelands.

For immigrants, assimilation into the American culture is not instantaneous, and, for adult immigrants, the process is never complete. In contrast, for their native-born children, and for those who arrive in the United States as young children, assimilation is a natural process that occurs with the inevitable immersion of these youth in American schools and culture. A large body of research shows that the children of immigrants do remarkably well in American schools, in part because immigrant parents push their children to excel by reminding them of their own sacrifices (Hirschman, 2014).

These high expectations for the children of immigrants generally lead to high motivations for academic and worldly success (Hao & Bonstead-Bruns, 1998). For example, several recent studies have found that foreign-born scientists and engineers are playing a critical role in American universities, laboratories, and scientific industries (Sana, 2010; Stephan & Levin, 2007), and that immigrants and their children are overrepresented in a broad range of rare achievements, including Nobel Prize winners, top scientists, American performing artists, and other contributors to the American creative arts.

Compared with other societies, the United States is generally regarded as unusually competitive and places a high premium on progress and innovation. This dynamic characteristic may well arise from the presence of immigrants and on the evolution of American institutions and identity because American institutions are meritocratic and seek the best talent wherever they can find it, pushing the country to value skills and ability over social pedigree. Over time, openness and the meritocratic processes may have become a force that shaped the evolution of American institutions in the arts, sports, science, and some sectors of business.

From the very origins of the nation and unlike many other societies, the United States does not have an identity tied to an ancient lineage. In spite of the historical contradiction and the stain of slavery, the American identity that was crafted by the founding fathers was based on the ideas of the *enlightment*. One of the country's founding fathers, Thomas Jefferson, argued that the group of individuals who would lead the destinies of the new nation would not be an aristocracy of lineage or blood, but an "aristocracy of virtue and talent, which nature has wisely provided for the direction of the interests of society, and scattered with equal hand through all its conditions," and that these human qualities would be "deemed essential to a well ordered republic" (Peterson, 1984). In turn, the five centuries of contributions by outsiders have reinforced a distinctive American character and culture that values not Who are you? but What can you do?

Currently, the overwhelming majority of the American population, including White Americans, is descended from nineteenth- and twentieth-century immigrants, so immigration is, perhaps, the most distinctive feature of the American identity. American history is largely the story of how immigrants have been absorbed into American society and how immigrants have enlarged and transformed America (Hirschman, 2014).

REFERENCES

Adelman, R., Reid, L. W., Markle, G., Weiss, S., & Jaret, C. (2017). Urban crime rates and the changing face of immigration: Evidence across four decades. *Journal of Ethnicity in Criminal Justice, 15*(1), 52–77. http://www.annualreviews.org/doi/abs/10.1146/annurev-criminol-032317-092026

Alba, R. D. (1990). *Ethnic identity: The transformation of White America.* New Haven, CT: Yale University Press.

American Psychiatric Association, Committee on Hispanic Psychiatrists. (2010). Position statement on xenophobia, immigration, and mental health. *American Journal of Psychiatry, 167,* 726.

Bar-Haim, Y., Ziv, T., Lamy, D., & Hodes, R. M. (2006). Nature and nurture in own-race face processing. *Psychological Science, 17,* 159–163.

Berry, J. W. (1997). Immigration, acculturation and adaptation. *Applied Psychology, 46*(1), 5–68.

Camarota, S. A., & Vaughan, J. M. (2009, November). Immigration and crime: Assessing a conflicted issue. Center for Immigration Studies. https://www.cis.org/sites/cis.org/files/articles/2009/crime.pdf

Chiao, J., Harada, T., Komeda, H., et al. (2009). Dynamic cultural influences on neural representations of the self. *Journal of Cognitive Neuroscience, 22,* 1–11.

Coatsworth, J. H. (2004). Globalization, growth and welfare in history. In M. M. Suarez-Orozco & D. Baolian Qin-Hilliard (Eds.), *Globalization, culture and education in the new millennium* (p. 1). Berkeley: University of California Press.

Cross, T., Bazron, B., Dennis, K., & Issac, M. (1989). *Towards a culturally competent system of care.* Washington, D.C.: CASSP Technical Assistance Center, Georgetown University Child Development Center.

Darwin, C. (1859). *On the origin of species by means of natural selection, or the preservation of favoured races in the struggle for life* (p. 502). London: Murray.

Derr, A. S. (2016). Mental health service use among immigrants in the United States: A systematic review. *Psychiatric Services, 67*(3), 267–274.

Devine, P. (1989). Stereotypes and prejudice: Their automatic and controlled components. *Journal of Personality and Social Psychology, 44,* 20–33.

Erikson, E. (1968) *Identity, youth, and crisis.* New York: Norton.

Escobar, J. I., & Vega, W. A. (2000). Mental health and immigration's three AAA's: Where are we and where do we go from here? *Journal of Nervous and Mental Disease, 188*(1), 736–740.

Hao, L., & Bonstead-Bruns, M. (1998). Parent-child differences in educational expectations and the academic achievement of immigrant and native students. *Sociology of Education, 71,* 175–198.

Hirschman, C. (2014). Immigration to the United States: Recent trends and future prospects. *Malaysian Journal of Economic Studies, 51*(1), 69–85. http://faculty.washington.edu/charles/new%20PUBS/A124.pdf

Hughes, C. C. (1993). Culture in clinical psychiatry. In A. C. Gaw (Ed.), *Culture, ethnicity and mental illness* (pp. 3–42). Washington, D.C.: Psychiatric Press.

Lee, J., & Bean, F. D. (2004). America's changing color lines: Immigration, race/ethnicity, and multiracial identification. *Annual Review of Sociology, 30*, 221–242.

McAdams, D. (2001). The Psychology of Life Stories. *Review of General Psychology, 5*(2), 100–122.

Ousey, G., & Kubrin, C. (2009). Exploring the connection between immigration and violent crime rates in U.S. cities, 1980–2000. *Social Problems, 56*, 447–473.

Ousey, G., & Kubrin, C. (2018). Immigration and crime: Assessing a contentious issue. *Annual Review of Criminology, 1*, 63–84. http://www.annualreviews.org/doi/abs/10.1146/annurev-criminol-032317-092026. Accessed January 7, 2018.

Passel, J., & Cohn, D. (2009). *A portrait of unauthorized immigrants in the United States*. Washington, D.C.: Pew Research Center. https://www.pewresearch.org/hispanic/2009/04/14/a-portrait-of-unauthorized-immigrants-in-the-united-states/

Peterson, M. D. (1984). *Thomas Jefferson: Writings: Autobiography. Notes on the State of Virginia. Public and private papers. Addresses. Letters*. New York: Library of America, Literary Classics of the United States.

Poland, W. (1977). Pilgrimage: Action and tradition in self analysis. *American Journal of Psychoanalysis, 25*(2), 399–416.

Portes, A., & Rumbaut, R. (2006). *Immigrant America: A portrait*. 3rd. ed. Berkeley: University of California Press.

Pumariega, A. J., & Joshi, S. (2010). Culture and development in children and youth. *Child and Adolescent Psychiatry Clinics of North America, 19*(4), 661–680.

Pumariega, A. J., Rothe, E.M., Mian, A., et al. (2013). Practice parameters for cultural competence in child psychiatric practice. *Journal of the American Academy of Child and Adolescent Psychiatry, 52*(12), 1101–1115.

Rodriguez, J. (2006). Color-blind ideology and the cultural appropriation of hip-hop. *Journal of Contemporary Ethnography, 35*(6), 645–668.

Rothe, E., Pumariega, A. J., & Sabagh, D. (2011). Identity and acculturation in immigrant and second generation adolescents. *Adolescent Psychiatry, 1*(1), 72–81.

Sana, M. (2010). Immigrants and Natives in U.S. science and engineering occupations, 1994–2006. *Demography, 47*, 801–820.

Schwartz, S. J., Montgomery, M. J., & Briones, E. (2006). The role of identity in acculturation among immigrant people: Theoretical propositions, empirical questions, and applied recommendations. *Human Development, 49*, 1–30.

Schwartz, S. J., Zamboanga, B. L., Weisskirch, R. S., & Wang, S. C. (2009). The relationships of personal and cultural identity to adaptive and maladaptive psychosocial functioning in emerging adults. *Journal of Social Psychology, 150*(1), 1–33.

Smith, J. P., & Edmonston, B. (1997). *The new Americans: Economic, demographic, and fiscal effects of immigration*. Washington, D.C.: National Academy Press.

Sohoni, D. (2006). The immigrant problem: Modern day nativism on the web. *Current Sociology, 54*, 827–850.

Sohoni, D., & Sohoni, T. W. P (2014). Perceptions of immigrant criminality: Crime and social boundaries. *The Sociological Quarterly, 55*, 49–71.

Spence, D. P. (1982). *Narrative truth and historical truth: Meaning and interpretation in psychoanalysis*. New York: Norton.

Stein, J. Y., & Tuval-Mashiash, R. (2014). Loneliness and isolation in life-stories of Israeli veterans of combat and captivity. *Psychological Trauma Theory Research Practice and Policy*. https://www.researchgate.net/publication/262639083_Loneliness_and_Isolation_in_Life-Stories_of_Israeli_Veterans_of_Combat_and_Captivity. Accessed March 4, 2018.

Stephan, P. F., & Levin, S. G. (2007). Striking the Mother Lode in Science: The Importance of Age, Place, and Time First Edition. https://www.amazon.com/Striking-Mother-Lode-Science-Importance/dp/0195064054

United Nations High Commissioner for Refugees (UNHCR). (2016). Global trends: Forced displacement in 2016. http://www.unhcr.org/5943e8a34.pdf. Accessed June 4, 2018.

Waters, M. C. (1990). *Ethnic options: Choosing identities in America*. Berkeley: University of California Press.

Zatz, M. S., & Smith, H. (2012). Immigration, crime and victimization: Rhetoric and reality. *Annual Review of Law and Social Science*, *8*, 141–159.

Zhu, Y., Zhang, L., Fan, J., & Han, S. (2007). Neural basis of cultural influence on self-representation. *NeuroImage*, *34*, 1310–1316.

INDEX

For the benefit of digital users, indexed terms that span two pages (e.g., 52–53) may, on occasion, appear on only one of those pages.